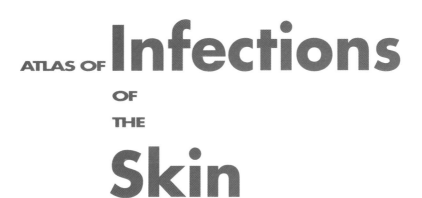

ATLAS OF Infections OF THE Skin

Anthony du Vivier

MD, FRCP

Department of Dermatology
King's College Hospital
London, UK

Gower Medical Publishing · LONDON · NEW YORK

Distributed in the USA and Canada by:
J B Lippincott Company
East Washington Square
Philadelphia
PA 19105
USA

Distributed in the UK and Continental
Europe by:
Gower Medical Publishing
Middlesex House
34–42 Cleveland Street
London W1P 5FB
UK

Distributed in Australia and New
Zealand by:
Harper and Row (Australia) Pty Ltd
PO Box 226
Artarmon
NSW 2064
Australia

Distributed in Southeast Asia, Hong
Kong, India and Pakistan by:
Harper and Row (Asia) Pte Ltd
37 Jalan Pemimpin 02-01
Singapore 2057

Distributed in Japan by:
Nankodo Co Ltd
42-6 Hongo 3-chome
Bunkyo-ku
Tokyo 113
Japan

British Library Cataloguing in Publication
Data:
du Vivier, Dr Anthony
    Atlas of infections of the skin.
    I. Title.
    616.5

Library of Congress Cataloging in
Publication Data:
du Viver, Anthony
    Atlas of infections of the skin / Anthony
    du Vivier.
    Includes index.
    1. Skin—Infections—Atlases. I. Title.
    [DNLM: 1. Skin Diseases, Infectious—
    atlases. WR 17 D987ab]
RL201.D8   1991
616.5—dc20

ISBN 0 397 44839 2

Publisher:
Fiona Foley

Project Manager:
Alison Whitehouse

Design and Layout:
Clare E. Gillmore
Pete Tex Wilder

Index:
Nina Boyd

Production:
Susan Bishop

Typesetting by J&L Composition Ltd,
Filey, North Yorkshire
Text set in Garamond; captions in Helvetica
Illustrations originated in Hong Kong by
Bright Arts Pte
Origination by Hilo Offset Limited,
Colchester
Produced by Mandarin Offset
Printed in Hong Kong

PREFACE

Infections of the skin are common. Some are easy to diagnose, such as warts and impetigo, but others, for example superficial fungal disorders and scabies, are more subtle. The latter are frequently misdiagnosed and consequently mistreated with topical steroids, which inevitably makes them worse. This book illustrates and discusses common bacteriological, fungal and viral infections of the skin; and also includes infestations. Less common disorders endemic to tropical countries, such as leprosy and leishmaniasis, are also described because the migration of populations and the ease of modern travel have made their appearance in the West more frequent.

Dermatological disorders are difficult to visualize mentally from simple textbook descriptions. It is therefore to be hoped that the wealth of illustrations in this book will complement the text and aid diagnosis. The *Atlas of Infections of the Skin* should be of interest to general practitioners, microbiologists and dermatologists, as well as to students.

Anthony du Vivier
London

ACKNOWLEDGEMENTS

The vast majority of the illustrations are, unless otherwise stated, of patients under the care of myself or members of the department of dermatology at King's College Hospital, London. The photographs have largely been taken by the medical illustration department of King's College Hospital or myself. The rest come from the photographic departments of the hospitals where I trained viz. St. Bartholomew's, St. Mary's and St. John's, London. I particularly wish to thank therefore Mr. E. Blewitt, Dr. D. Tredinnick, Dr. P. Cardew, Mr. B. Pike, Mr. E. Sparkes and Mr. S. Robertson and their departments for the help they have given me over the years.

I wish also to acknowledge with deep gratitude the physicians who have taught me dermatology and influenced me. They are Drs. Dowling Munro, Julian Verbov, Michael Feiwel, Richard Stoughton, Gerald Levene, Eugene van Scott, Peter Samman, Bob Marten, Professor Malcolm Greaves and the late Dr. Peter Borrie.

I am indebted to Dr. Phillip McKee for his help regarding the biology and pathology of diseases of the skin included in this atlas and to Drs. Andrew Pembroke and Jeremy Gilkes, my colleagues, for their advice and support.

Finally the atlas is dedicated to my wife, Judith, who makes everything worthwhile.

All histopathology transparencies have been provided by Dr. Phillip McKee unless otherwise stated.

CONTENTS

1

Bacterial Infections of the Skin

IMPETIGO

This is a superficial cutaneous infection caused by either *Staphylococcus aureus* or a β-haemolytic streptococcus or both. It is particularly common in children and adolescents. The condition is highly contagious and will spread rapidly in any institution such as a boarding school or a nursery. The primary lesion is a vesicle or blister (Fig. 1.1) containing yellow pus (Fig. 1.2). It extends, becoming circinate or polycyclic (Fig. 1.3) before rupturing, and produces a yellow, honey-coloured crust (Fig. 1.4).

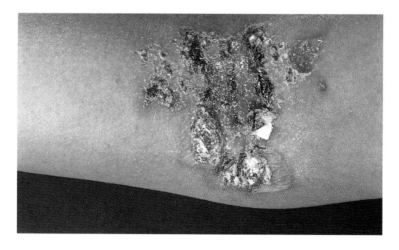

Fig. 1.1 Impetigo. The lesions start as blisters which contain pus and subsequently become eroded and crusted.

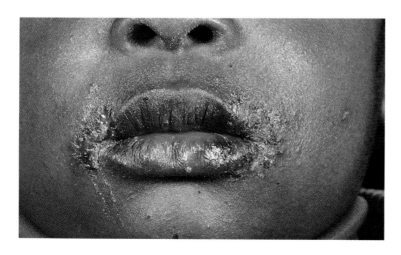

Fig. 1.2 Impetigo. The lesions ooze pus.

The lesions occur most often on the face (Fig. 1.5), but may be found anywhere on the skin. The condition is an acute one and autoinoculation causes it to spread to other sites. It most frequently arises

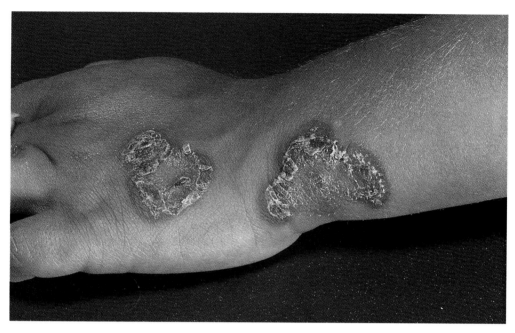

Fig. 1.3 Impetigo. The lesions may be polycyclic and heal centrally.

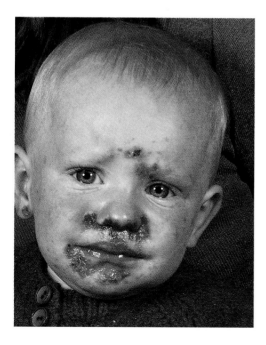

Fig. 1.4 Impetigo. The face is a common site. Golden crusts are present. Infants and children are particularly at risk.

de novo although predisposing causes, such as infestation and, in particular, pediculosis capitis or eczema (Fig. 1.6) may be present. Treatment with the appropriate antibiotic either topically or, more often, systemically will result in resolution of the condition within a day or so. Many staphylococcal infections

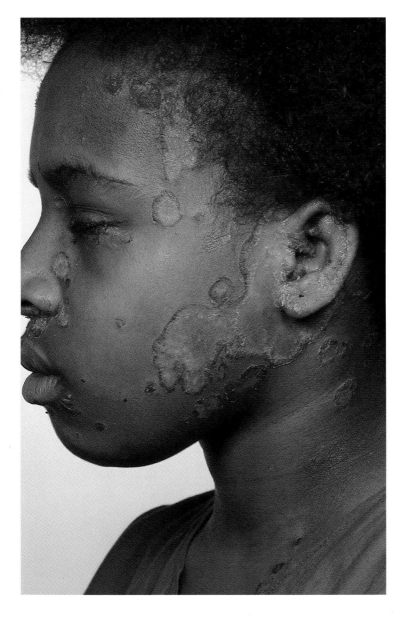

Fig. 1.5 Impetigo. The lesions may spread rapidly especially if topical steroids are inappropriately prescribed.

are resistant to penicillin so erythromycin is the usual choice of antibiotic. The streptococcal infections are sensitive to penicillin but also to erythromycin.

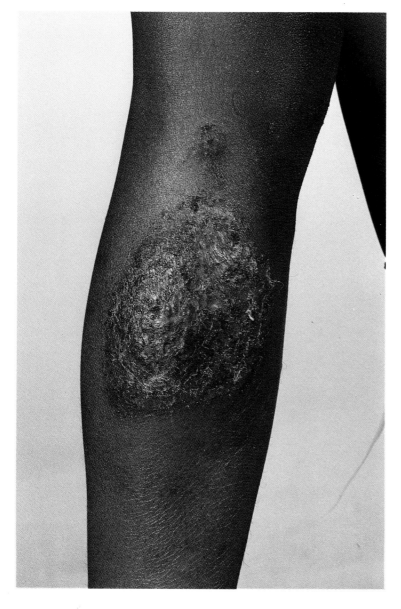

Fig. 1.6 Impetiginized eczema. Impetigo may occur as a secondary event. Eczema often becomes infected and yellow brown crusting results.

FOLLICULITIS

When correctly used, this term implies a superficial bacterial infection of the hair follicle. However, it is also used to describe sterile, follicular pustules from which pathogenic bacteria can not be recovered and which probably would be better classified as pseudofolliculitis.

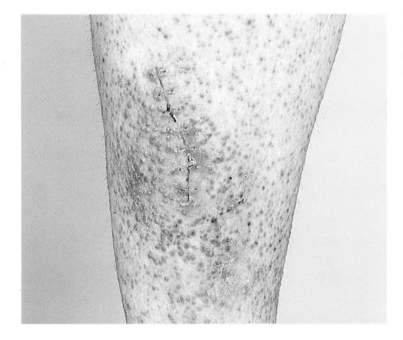

Fig. 1.7 Folliculitis. Septic pustules have occurred under an occlusive dressing following a leg operation.

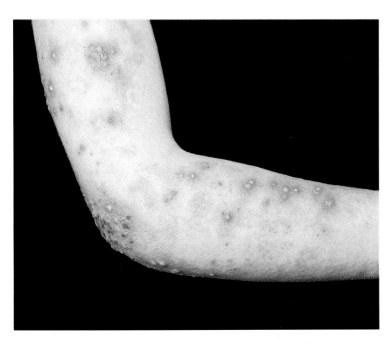

Fig. 1.8 Folliculitis. Discrete yellow pustules surrounded by erythema are a common complication of topical glucorticosteroid treatment of skin disorders. By courtesy of St. John's Hospital for Diseases of the Skin.

Bockhart's Impetigo

This is an acute, staphylococcal or streptococcal infection of the skin, seen particularly on the lower limbs of hirsute individuals (Fig. 1.7). It is also fairly common in patients using topical glucocorticosteroids for eczema and psoriasis (Fig. 1.8). Small, discrete, painful, yellow, follicular pustules are evident. The condition responds rapidly to appropriate systemic antibiotics.

Sycosis Barbae

This is a chronic deep-seated staphylococcal infection of the beard area (Fig. 1.9). It is only seen in men and is now very rare in Western societies, probably as a result of better hygienic conditions and the widespread availability and early use of antibiotics. There is, however, a common condition caused by ingrowing hairs which is frequently misnamed sycosis barbae.

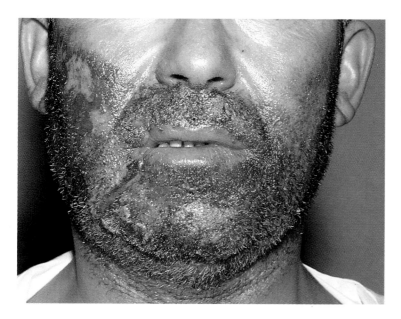

Fig. 1.9 Sycosis barbae. Staphylococcal infection of the beard area is uncommon in Western societies probably because of improved hygiene and early use of antibiotics.

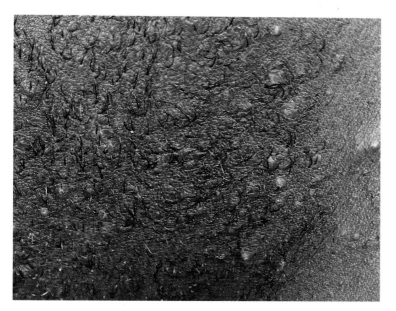

Fig. 1.10 Folliculitis secondary to ingrowing hairs. A sterile acneiform eruption develops secondary to ingrowing hairs. It is particularly common in negroes.

Folliculitis Secondary to Ingrowing Hairs

This condition is found commonly, but not exclusively, in negroes. The hairs in the beard area, particularly under the jaw, tend to grow back into the skin resulting in an acneiform, follicular, pustular eruption (Fig. 1.10). In negroes, this may result in keloid formation (Figs. 1.11 and 1.12). The disorder responds poorly to antibiotics although there may be a marginal response to long-term, low-dose antibiotics given in a similar manner as in the treatment of acne vulgaris. The condition can, however, be resolved by growing a beard, although this is not always acceptable.

Folliculitis of the Scalp

This is relatively common in negroes where yellow pustules are seen surrounding the hairs. Although *Staphylococcus aureus* is readily cultured from the lesions, the condition is not eradicated by treating with

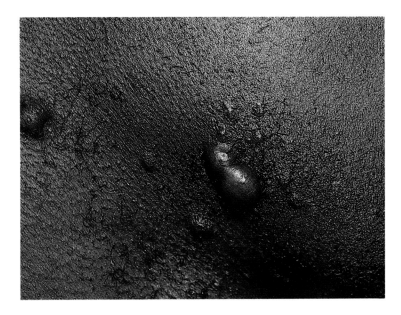

Fig. 1.11 Keloids secondary to folliculitis. Keloids may result from the pseudofolliculitis associated with ingrowing hairs.

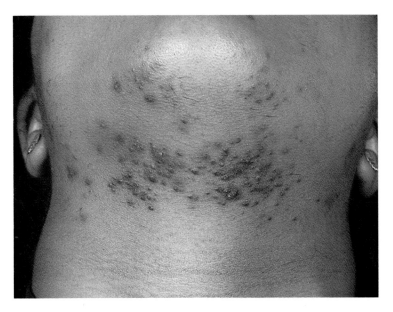

Fig. 1.12 Keloids secondary to ingrowing hairs in hirsute female.

the appropriate antibiotic. It tends to be recalcitrant and chronic with fresh lesions developing all the time and may well result in considerable keloid formation, particularly at the back of the neck (Fig. 1.13).

Pseudomonas Folliculitis

Outbreaks of folliculitis have been reported in the United States since 1975, secondary to the use of contaminated whirlpools. Pustules develop on the torso and limbs (Fig. 1.14) within 24–48 hours of exposure. *Pseudomonas aeruginosa* may be cultured from the pustules. The patient may be unwell with malaise and low-grade fever and lympadenopathy. Otitis externa, mastitis, ocular and urinary tract infections may also occur. Whirlpools are much more prone to contamination than swimming pools, partly because of difficulties in maintaining adequate chlorination of the water. The chlorine evaporates easily due to the high temperatures and continual agitation of the water by the pressurized jets of the jacuzzi. There is usually a high concentration of organic matter which encourages the growth of the bacteria and tends to reduce the chlorine to less-active forms. The heat of the water also dilates the follicular openings and facilitates the entry of the bacteria. The condition is self-limiting and the patient recovers in a week or ten days without treatment.

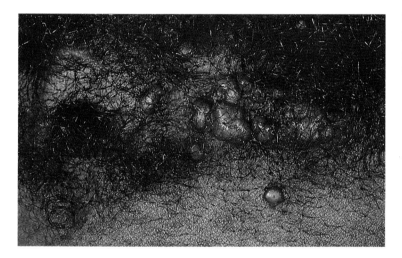

Fig. 1.13 Nuchal keloids. Folliculitis of the scalp often results in keloids especially at the back of the neck.

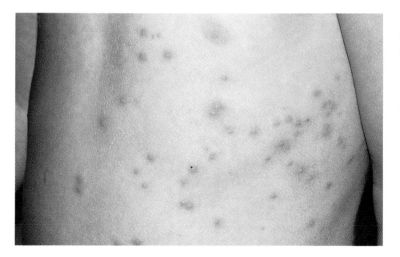

Fig. 1.14 Pseudomonas folliculitis. Widespread pustules surrounded by erythema may develop from the use of jacuzzis contaminated with *Pseudomonas aeruginosa*.

Folliculitis due to Acne and Oils

Sterile follicular pustules are common on the limbs, particularly the thighs, of individuals who have a tendency to acne and are hirsute. Those who wear tight, occlusive clothing or have an occupation where there clothes become contaminated with oil (Figs. 1.15 and 1.16) are prone to this kind of folliculitis.

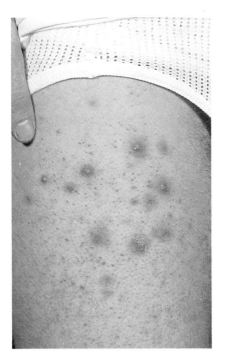

Fig. 1.15 Folliculitis due to oils. Sterile acneiform papules and pustules develop secondary to follicular occlusion due to oils.

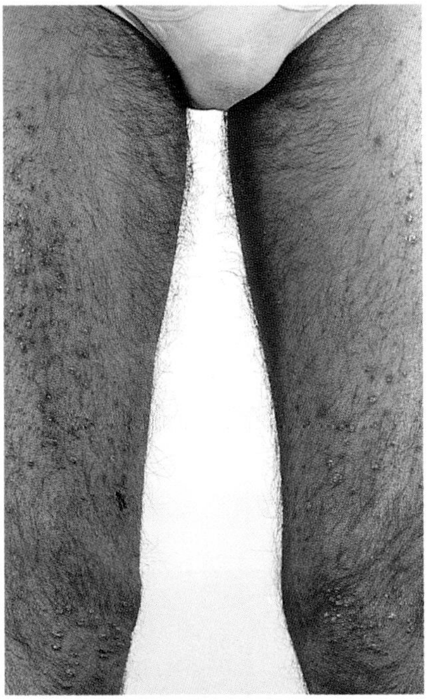

Fig. 1.16 Folliculitis due to oils. Hirsutism predisposes to this condition. The thighs are a common site particularly if oily tight-fitting trousers are worn. By courtesy of Dr. A.C. Pembroke.

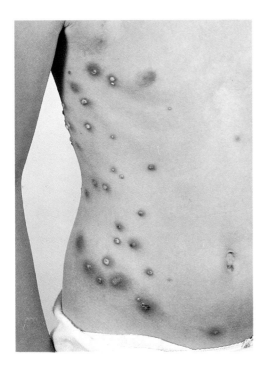

Fig. 1.17 Furunculosis (boils). Painful red nodules are present in various stages of development.

FURUNCULOSIS (Boils)

This is an acute staphylococcal infection of the hair follicles (Fig. 1.17). It differs from folliculitis in that there is a greater degree of inflammation and the infection spreads away from the hair follicle into the surrounding dermis. Pus may become visible on the surface of the lesion as it evolves (Fig. 1.18) and will discharge either spontaneously or as a result of lancing. A deep abscess may leave scarring (Fig. 1.19). A carbuncle is a collection of boils such that multiple draining sites occur. The patient is usually unwell and has a fever. The condition responds rapidly to appropriate antibiotics. Occasionally, however, boils may become recurrent. In these cases the patient is usually a chronic carrier of staphylococci, either in the anterior nares, perineum or axillae, often acquired after a period of hospitalization. Swabs should be taken from these sites and the carrier sites treated with topical antibiotics for several weeks. It may be necessary to take an additional prolonged course of antibiotics, and also it is useful to sterilize the skin by adding hexachlorophane to the daily bath.

Although always recorded in textbooks, it is rare that a patient presenting with boils proves to have previously unsuspected diabetes mellitus, but it is routine practice to test the urine for glycosuria. Occasionally, immunosuppressed patients may present with boils.

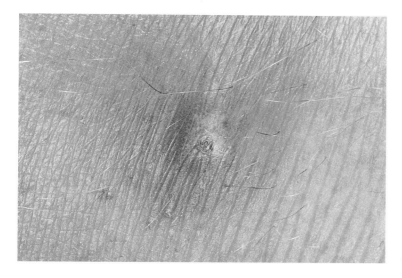

Fig. 1.18 Furunculosis. The pus is pointing on the surface of this red tender module.

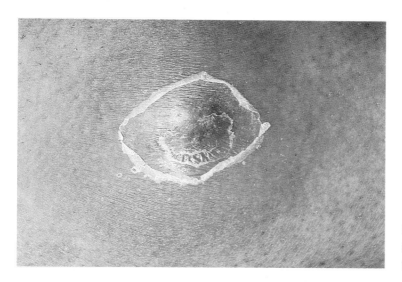

Fig. 1.19 Furunculosis. As the boil expands there is a peeling of the overlying skin.

STYES (Hordeoli)

A stye is a staphylococcal infection of an eyelash (Fig. 1.20) and has the same clinical features as a boil although it is much smaller in size. Many affected patients also carry the staphylococcus in their anterior nares, which should also be treated. Chronic staphylococcal infections of the eyelashes occasionally occur (Fig. 1.21).

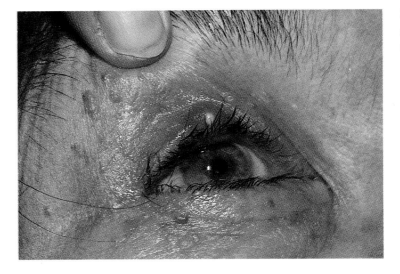

Fig.1.20 Stye. This is an acute staphylococcal infection of an eyelash. The pus is pointing.

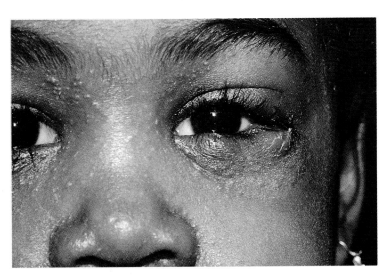

Fig. 1.21 Chronic sepsis of the eyelashes. Chronic staphylococcal infections may be associated with carriage of the bacteria in the nose.

ECTHYMA

This is a bacterial infection of the skin caused by either *Staphylococcus aureus* or streptococci. It begins in a similar way to impetigo (as a superficial vesicle containing pus) but extends more deeply and enters the dermis. The condition presents as crusted ulcers, particularly on the lower legs (Fig. 1.22). It is a common consequence of insect bites and particularly occurs in hot countries. It presented particular problems to American troops in Vietnam.

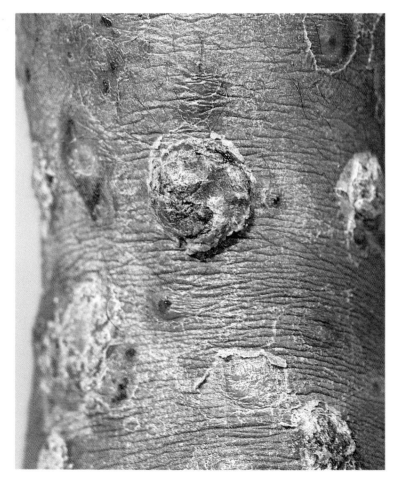

Fig. 1.22 Ecthyma. Crusted and eroded lesions present mainly on the lower legs. Insect bites are the most common cause and sepsis results. By courtesy of St. Mary's Hospital.

TOXIC EPIDERMAL NECROLYSIS ('Scalded Skin' Syndrome)

This is an uncommon condition of children, particularly of the very young. Early recognition of the disease and treatment with appropriate antibiotics may be life-saving. It is caused by an epidermolytic toxin, usually produced by a Group 2 staphylococcus, phage type 71. It appears to be an individual

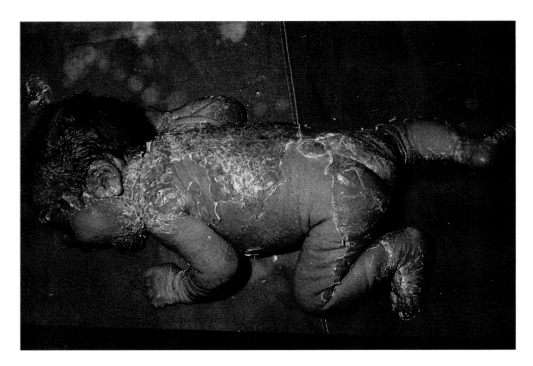

Fig. 1.23 Scalded skin syndrome (Lyell's syndrome). Epidermal necrolysis occurs secondary to staphylococcal toxin. The skin may be universally red and desquamating resembling a burn.

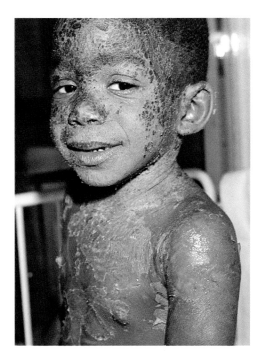

Fig. 1.24 Scalded skin syndrome. The skin becomes raw and eroded. The similarity to impetigo is clear. The condition responds rapidly to antibiotics.

idiosyncratic response since other members of the same family may have staphylococcal infection which is manifest only as impetigo. A most characteristic symptom is extreme tenderness of the skin followed shortly by redness and widespread desquamation of the epidermis in sheets (Fig. 1.23). This reveals red, raw and eroded skin resembling a superficial burn (Fig. 1.24). Most, or all, of the body surface may be involved with the desquamation. A similar eruption occurs in adults, but this is drug-induced and not caused by a staphylococcus and does not respond to antibiotics. The histopathology of the staphylococcal 'scalded skin' syndrome reveals the damage to be superficial, in the granular cell layer, whereas in drug-induced disease the damage is in the region of the dermo-epidermal junction.

ERYSIPELAS

This is an acute, superficial infection of the skin, normally caused by streptococcus. The condition is sometimes known as 'St. Anthony's fire'. The clinical distinction of erysipelas from cellulitis is often difficult; erysipelas is more superficial and usually affects the face (Fig. 1.25), while cellulitis also affects the subcutaneous tissue. Cellulitis may also be caused by staphylococcus, usually involving the lower leg.

The onset of the condition is sudden. The patient is ill, has a high fever and rigors, may vomit and become quite delirious. Examination reveals a unilateral eruption, occurring either on one leg or on one side of the face or scalp. The area involved is sharply delineated, red and tender (Fig. 1.26) and there is associated oedema and sometimes blistering (Fig. 1.27) and erosions (Fig. 1.28). The condition responds dramatically to appropriate antibiotic therapy although the patient may be left with a persistent oedema of the lower leg.

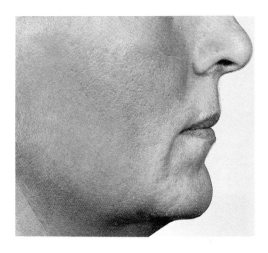

Fig. 1.25 Erysipelas. There is erythema and oedema usually unilaterally. The onset is sudden. The patient feels ill and may have a rigor.

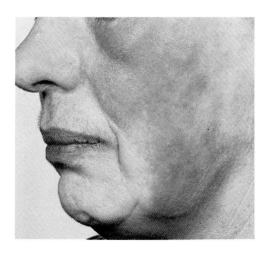

Fig. 1.26 Erysipelas. Recurrent attacks are common probably due to lymphatic deficiency. Continual low dose antibiotic therapy usually prevents further episodes.

It is thought that the organism penetrates the skin via a breach in the epidermis. On the face, this may be difficult to identify but on the leg there is often associated tinea pedis. The condition may become recurrent, probably due to a relative deficiency of lymphatics. This lymphatic hypoplasia may be present primarily or result from the erysipelas. Recurrent attacks should be treated with long-term antibiotics. Small doses of penicillin or erythromycin taken daily are often very effective. Associated predisposing causes such as otitis externa or tinea pedis should be treated.

LYMPHANGIITIS

This is an inflammation of the subcutaneous lymphatic channels secondary to infection, usually by a streptococcus. It presents as linear red streaks ön the skin (Fig. 1.29) associated with tender regional lymphadenopathy. It responds to treatment of the source of the infection.

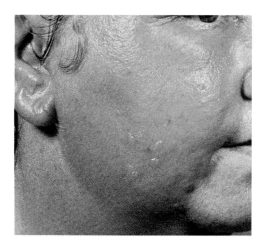

Fig. 1.27 Erysipelas. There may be blistering in addition to the erythema and oedema.

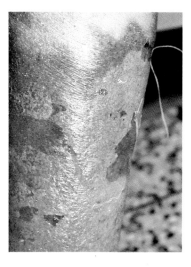

Fig. 1.28 Erysipelas. Erosions may follow erythema, oedema and blistering. The lower leg is a common site.

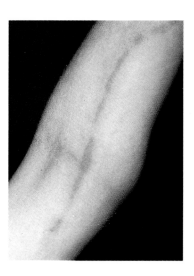

Fig. 1.29 Lymphangiitis. A linear red streak has resulted from an infected conditon of the hand. Lymphadenopathy is usually present.

ERYSIPELOID

This is an uncommon infection with the Gram-positive bacteria *Erysipelothrix rhusiopathiae*. It occurs in those whose occupation includes handling contaminated raw fish or meat. The organism enters the skin through an abrasion and is most likely to be seen on the hand. Erysipeloid involves a slowly evolving process lasting a few weeks and consisting of a purple to red, slightly oedematous eruption (Fig. 1.30) with a well-defined, raised edge which spreads over the fingers, with a tendency to heal at its original site. Unlike erysipelas, there is no systemic disturbance. It responds to treatment with penicillin.

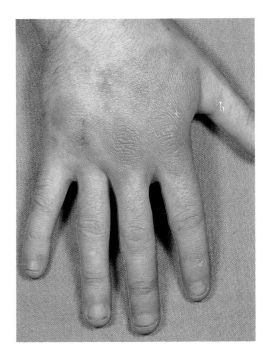

Fig. 1.30 Erysipeloid. Erythema and oedema are present on the back of the hand. By courtesy of St. Mary's Hospital.

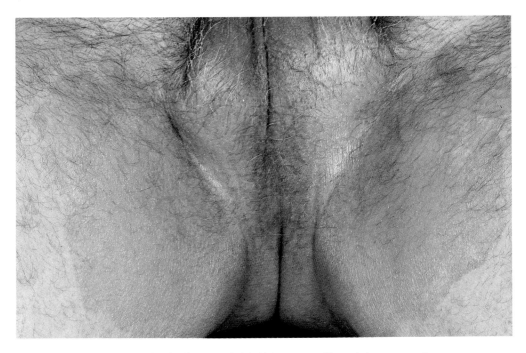

Fig. 1.31 Erythrasma. A brown discoloration occurs in intertriginous areas. The groin is a common site.

ERYTHRASMA

This is a bacterial infection of the skin caused by *Corynebacterium minutissimum*. The disease causes an intertrigo and is most common in the groins (Fig. 1.31), axillae (Fig. 1.32) or under the breasts. It causes a well-defined brown discoloration (Figs. 1.33 and 1.34) with a fine wrinkled, slightly scaly surface. It fluoresces a coral-pink colour under Wood's light and this aids the diagnosis (Fig. 1.35). It is often present as maceration of the skin between the toes, and is more common in those who live in hot countries. It responds to topical imidazoles or oral erythromycin.

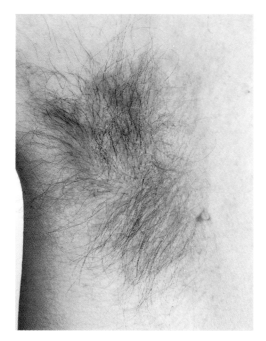

Fig. 1.32 Erythrasma. The axillae are commonly involved. The condition is more common in hot climates.

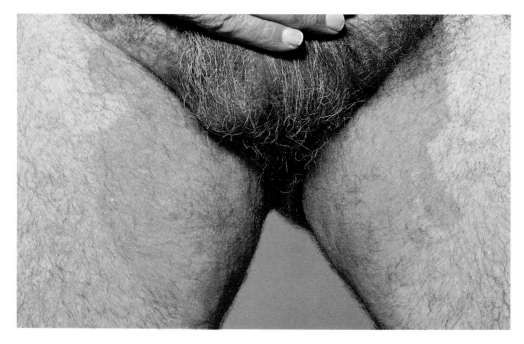

Fig. 1.33 Erythrasma. The discoloration is caused by *Corynebacterium minutissimum*. By courtesy of St. Mary's Hospital.

TUBERCULOSIS OF THE SKIN

Cutaneous tuberculosis is becoming increasingly uncommon in Western countries following the advent of drugs which can successfully combat the disease and reduce the foci of infection and also as a result of improvements in the nutritional and economic state of the community. The type of lesion produced in the skin depends on whether or not the patient has acquired any immunity to the disease in the past. There is thus both primary tuberculosis of the skin and so-called 'post-primary' disease. In addition, there are cutaneous reactions to the presence of tuberculosis elsewhere in the body which are known as tuberculides.

Primary Tuberculosis of the Skin

Susceptible individuals are those who have never had a previous infection with *Mycobacterium tuberculosis*. The Mantoux test is negative. Direct inoculation of the bacilli into the skin produces a chancre with associated lymphadenitis. The chancre starts as a brown papule which frequently ulcerates and persists as a sore. The edge of the ulcer may be undermined with an adherent crust on the surface. It may occur anywhere on the body but since the bacilli are thought to be introduced via traumatized skin it is usually seen on exposed parts such as the face or limbs, particularly in children.

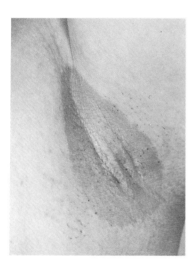

Fig. 1.34 Erythrasma. A brown discoloration is present in the axillae.

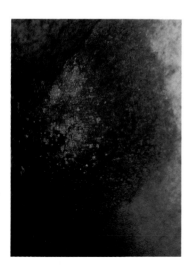

Fig. 1.35 Erythrasma. The organism fluoresces a coral-pink colour under a Wood's light. By courtesy of Dr. Y.M. Clayton, St. John's Hospital for Diseases of the Skin.

BCG Granuloma

A similar lesion to the above may occur after BCG vaccination of an already immune individual (Figs. 1.36 and 1.37). Biopsy of the lesion reveals a granulomatous histology and acid-fast bacilli are demonstrable on Ziehl–Neelsen staining of the section.

Lupus Vulgaris

This variety of cutaneous tuberculosis results from lymphatic or haematogenous spread from a focus in a bone, joint or lymph node. There is usually a solitary lesion on the face (Fig. 1.38), neck or on a limb. It is a red-brown, somewhat raised, well-demarcated plaque (Fig. 1.39). By pressing the lesion with a glass slide (a procedure known as diascopy) small nodules within the plaque appear as a translucent brown colour, somewhat reminiscent of apple jelly. Subsequently the epidermis overlying the dermal

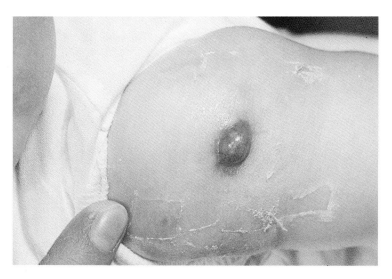

Fig. 1.36 BCG vaccination. A solitary brown nodule is present at the site of BCG vaccination against tuberculosis. The child had had no previous exposure to the disease.

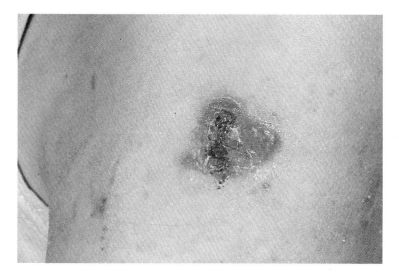

Fig. 1.37 BCG granuloma. The lesion ulcerates and persists as a sore.

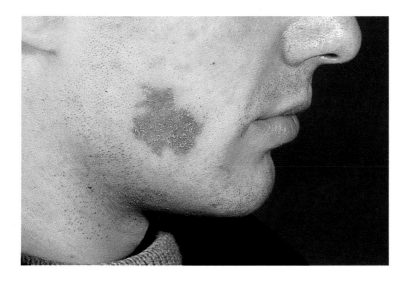

Fig. 1.38 Lupus vulgaris. There is a solitary plaque on the face. The cheek is the commonest site.

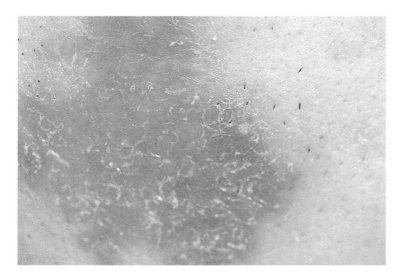

Fig. 1.39 Lupus vulgaris. The plaque has an 'apple jelly' colour and scaling is present.

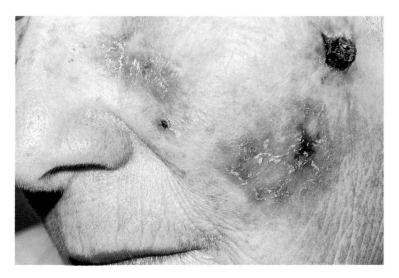

Fig. 1.40 Lupus vulgaris. The skin becomes atrophic and scarred.

granuloma becomes scaly and atrophic (Fig. 1.40). Superficial ulceration and scarring may result. Similar lesions may occur on a limb (Figs. 1.41 and 1.42). Biopsy of the skin confirms the diagnosis (Fig. 1.43). The condition should clear with appropriate anti-tuberculosis therapy but occasionally the disorder is chronic. After many decades there is a risk of squamous cell carcinoma developing in the lesion.

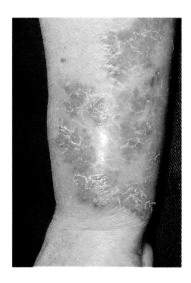

Fig. 1.41 Lupus vulgaris. The brown colour is very typical of lupus on this woman's arm.

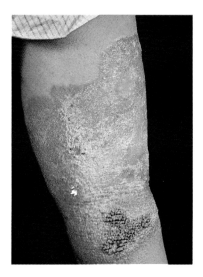

Fig. 1.42 Lupus vulgaris. The lesion is raised, well-demarcated and warty. Skin biopsy for culture and histology can easily be performed.

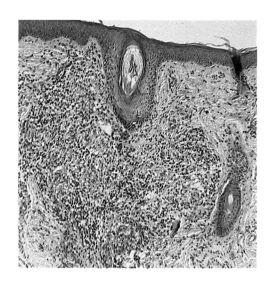

Fig. 1.43 Lupus vulgaris. An ill-defined granulomatous infiltrate containing giant cells is situated in the upper dermis, in close proximity to a hair follicle. There is a heavy admixture of lymphocytes and caseation necrosis is absent. Such features although not absolutely diagnostic are highly suggestive of lupus vulgaris. As is often the case, a Ziehl–Neelsen stain for tubercle bacilli was negative.

Tuberculosis Verrucosa Cutis

This is a rare condition secondary to direct inoculation of tubercle bacilli into the skin (Fig. 1.44), usually through an abrasion in a person whose occupation might involve handling material contaminated with the bacilli. Thus, butchers can contract the disease from animals ('butcher's warts') and pathologists from humans during post-mortem examinations. The lesion is usually single and consists of a hyperkeratotic warty plaque on a hand or limb. The red-brown colour of the lesion is suggestive of the diagnosis but a skin biopsy is mandatory. This should confirm the diagnosis.

Scrofuloderma

This term refers to direct infection of tubercle bacilli from an underlying infected lymph node (Fig. 1.45) or bone to the skin. The side of the neck, supraclavicular fossa or axillae are common sites. There is a fluctuant swelling which suppurates and ulcerates. The condition heals on treatment but leaves considerable scarring.

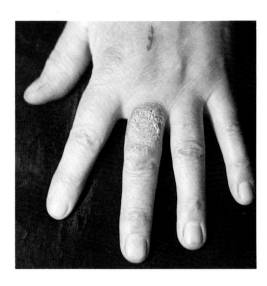

Fig. 1.44 Tuberculosis verrucosa cutis. This condition results from direct inoculation of tubercle bacilli into the skin. It usually occurs as a solitary lesion in a person whose occupation could entail handling contaminated material. By courtesy of St. John's Hospital for Diseases of the Skin.

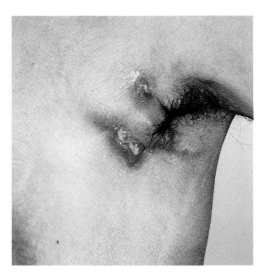

Fig. 1.45 Scrofuloderma. Direct extension to the skin has resulted from infected lymph nodes in the axillae.

Tuberculides

These are cutaneous immunological reactions to tuberculosis elsewhere in the individual, but no tubercle bacilli are demonstrable in the skin lesions.

Erythema Induratum (Bazin's Disease)

These skin lesions are essentially similar to those of erythema nodosum but they may ulcerate, unlike erythema nodosum, and they particularly affect the calves (Fig. 1.46) rather than the shins. The condition is probably the result of circulating immune complexes. The patient complains of painful swellings on the legs. There may be a concomitant fever and joint pains. On examination, red, tender, warm swellings are seen. Nodules can also occur on the fronts of the shins, ankles and feet and occasionally even on the

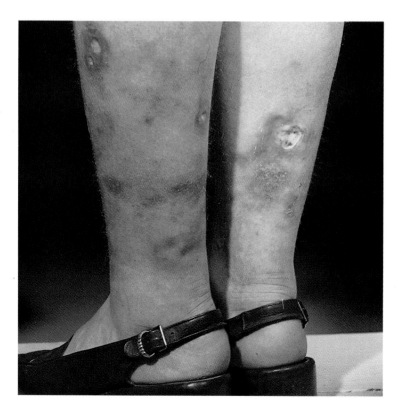

Fig. 1.46 Bazin's disease. Ulcerated tender nodules on the calves are suggestive of tuberculosis.

upper limbs. Erythema nodosum or erythema induratum are indications to search for evidence of tuberculosis elsewhere. The eruptions will respond to anti-tuberculous therapy. Occasionally no focus of tuberculosis is found in erythema induratum and yet the Mantoux test may be strongly positive. This particular variety does, however, respond to anti-tuberculous treatment.

Papulonecrotic Tuberculide

This is a rare condition occurring predominantly in young individuals who have active tuberculosis elsewhere. There is an eruption of necrotic, inflammatory, indolent papules which occur in crops on the extremities (Fig. 1.47). This is thought to be an immunological reaction. The histopathology is suggestive of a granuloma but no bacilli can be demonstrated in the lesions. The condition responds to the treatment of the tuberculosis elsewhere.

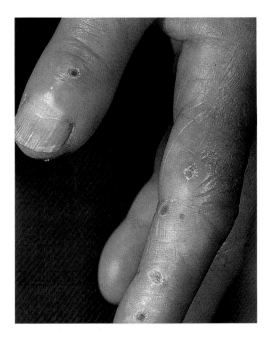

Fig. 1.47 Papulonecrotic tuberculide. Crops of necrotic indolent papules occur particularly on the extremities.

FISH-TANK AND SWIMMING POOL GRANULOMA

This infection is caused by *Mycobacterium marinum*. It is contracted from contaminated water via a skin abrasion. Fish-tanks or swimming pools are the usual sources. The patient may give a history of having cut the skin whilst cleaning out a fish-tank that previously housed diseased fish (Fig. 1.48). Alternatively, the patient may have abraded the skin of the face or a limb in a contaminated swimming pool. Purple-red nodules (Fig. 1.49) develop at the site of the injury and may subsequently appear along the line of lymphatic drainage from the inoculation site. Healing usually occurs spontaneously after a number of weeks or months.

The diagnosis is made by skin biopsy which shows a granulomatous histopathology. *Mycobacterium marinum* (syn. *balnei*) causes tuberculosis in fish. It is an acid-fast bacillus which can be grown on culture but must be incubated at 31°C and not the usual 37°C required for human tuberculosis.

There is no really specific treatment but success has been reported with rifampicin, septrin and minocycline.

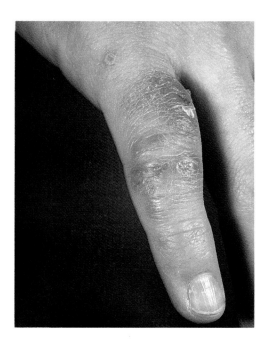

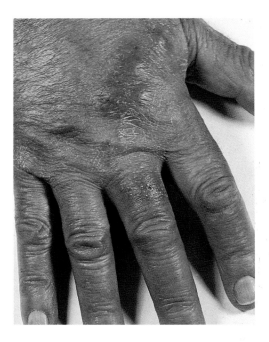

Fig. 1.48 Fish-tank granuloma. This young man had cut his skin on a fish-tank which he was cleaning. The tank had previously housed fish which had died of *Mycobacterium marinum*. By courtesy of St. Bartholomew's Hospital.

Fig. 1.49 Fish-tank granuloma. This man has developed purple nodules at the site of abrasions acquired whilst cleaning a fish-tank.

GONOCOCCAEMIA

Disseminated gonococcal infections may occur in untreated patients with gonorrhoea. They occur more commonly in females. The organism appears to be slightly different from that causing gonococcal urethritis, which remains limited to the mucous membranes.

The condition essentially affects the skin and the joints, although occasionally a pericarditits or meningitis occurs. The patient is unwell and feverish. The skin lesions are vesicles or pustules on an erythematous base (Fig. 1.50) and are found on the extremities, particularly the fingers (Fig. 1.51). They are sparse. The knees, wrists and ankles are the joints most commonly involved and often only one joint is affected.

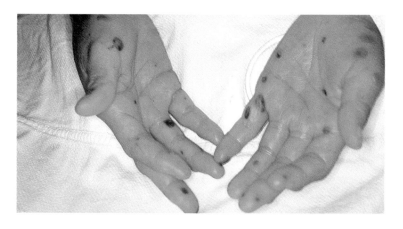

Fig. 1.50 Gonococcaemia. The lesions are haemorrhagic pustules on an erythematous base. By courtesy of Dr. Frank Dann, Honolulu.

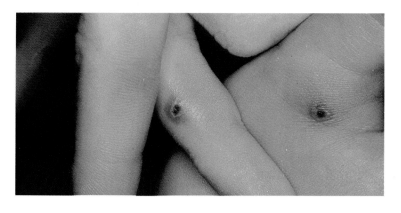

Fig. 1.51 Gonococcaemia. The extremities, particularly the hands, are affected. By courtesy of Dr. Frank Dann, Honolulu.

SYPHILIS

Syphilis is an infection with the spirochaete *Treponema pallidum*. Spirochaetes are thin-walled, flexible, helical rods. They have some features in common with bacteria but are unusual in that their mobility is due to an internal axial filament rather than the external flagella used by other mobile bacteria. Syphilis is usually transmitted sexually, particularly among homosexual men but may be acquired from maternal disease *in utero* or from infected blood products or instruments. The disease is divided into stages known as primary, secondary, latent and tertiary. The former two stages are infectious. If the disease is untreated, it may progress through all four stages or remit.

Primary Syphilis

The primary lesion or chancre occurs at the site of inoculation between ten days and three months after infection. It is thus usually on the genitalia or around the anus, but may occur elsewhere on the body, particularly on the lips, inside the mouth or rectum or on a finger. The chancre is a painless ulcer with an indurated edge (Fig. 1.52). The base is yellow and harbours a large number of spirochaetes which may be demonstrated by dark ground microscopy. The local lymph nodes are enlarged but are quite painless. The chancre heals spontaneously, often without trace, within one to three months.

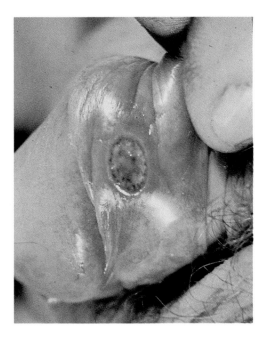

Fig. 1.52 Primary syphilis. The lesion is a painless ulcer with an indurated edge. The base is yellow and harbours large numbers of spirochaetes. By courtesy of Dr. F. Lim, King's College Hospital.

Secondary Syphilis

Most patients are diagnosed during the primary stage. However, if the chancre is not visible to the patient, either around the anus or in the rectum, the disease may evolve to the secondary stage. This occurs about two months after the chancre.

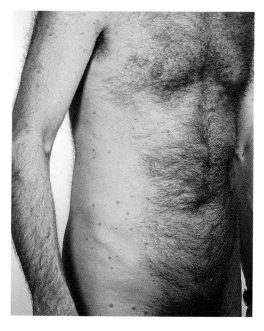

Fig. 1.53 Secondary syphilis. Initially the rash is macular and pink and is most obvious on the trunk. It does not itch. The serology is positive at this stage.

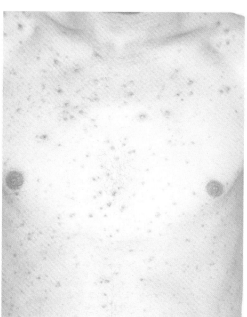

Fig. 1.54 Secondary syphilis. The lesions become papular and more widespread. There is a tendency towards cropping of the lesions. By courtesy of St. Mary's Hospital.

The patient usually has a fever and presents because of a rash. The eruption is widespread (Figs. 1.53 and 1.54) and particularly involves the genitalia (Figs. 1.55 and 1.56), palms and soles (Fig. 1.57) and face (Fig. 1.58). It does not itch although clearly if there is some complicating factor such as hepatitis or a second sexually acquired disease such as scabies, the skin will be pruritic. There is a generalized lymphadenopathy. The primary lesion may still be visible.

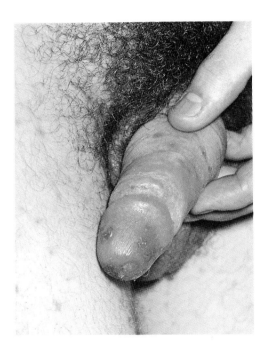

Fig. 1.55 Secondary syphilis. The genitalia are usually involved. By courtesy of St. Mary's Hospital.

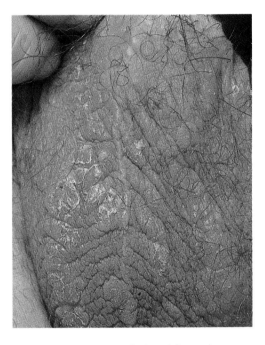

Fig. 1.56 Secondary syphilis. Scaly, red, firm patches are present on the scrotum.

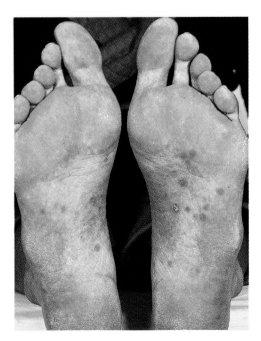

Fig. 1.57 Secondary syphilis. The soles (and palms) are invariably affected with papules.

Initially the rash is macular and pink (roseolar) and is most obvious on the trunk. It becomes papular and more widespread. There is a tendency to cropping of lesions. The papules become brown and may resemble pityriasis rosea or psoriasis. Later lesions may become more infiltrated (Fig. 1.59). The lesions may be more profuse around the frontal hair margin (crown of Venus) and sides of the neck (collar of Venus). Genital and palmar/plantar involvement are constant features. In the intertriginous areas the papules may be eroded (condylomata lata). Condylomata usually occur around the anus or in the groin but may occur under the axillae or breasts, in the umbilicus or between the toes. These lesions are usually moist and exude treponemes in the serum; they are therefore highly infectious.

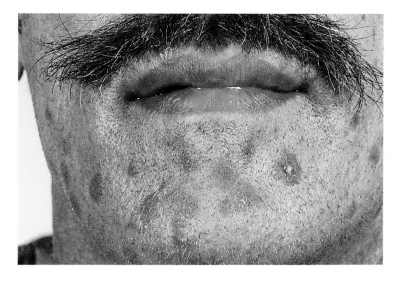

Fig. 1.58 Secondary syphilis. The face is usually involved. The papules may become scaly and resemble pityriasis rosea or psoriasis. Indeed, syphilis tends to mimic other diseases. This is the same patient as in Fig. 1.53.

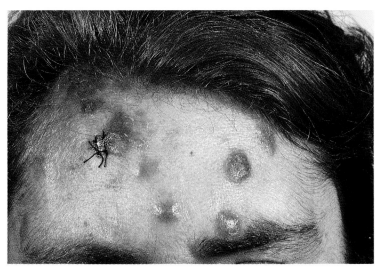

Fig. 1.59 Secondary syphilis. In the later stages, infiltrated plaques may develop. The brown colour of the lesions is characteristic. A skin biopsy was necessary and the histology suggested the diagnosis. Syphilis is uncommon in women; this woman's husband was bisexual.

Slightly raised oval patches occur on the mucous membranes (Fig. 1.60). The tongue, buccal mucous membranes, soft palate and fauces are most usually involved. The lesions have an off-white surface membrane. Several contiguous lesions are known as 'snail-track' ulcers.

Hair loss is common, either as part of the cutaneous eruption (Fig. 1.61) or subsequently as a telogen effluvium response to the systemic upset.

The patient may not be ill at all, but most have some degree of malaise. Headache, sore throat, hoarseness, deafness, photophobia, neck stiffness, polyarthritis and nocturnal bone pains may all occur. There may also be hepatitis and renal involvement. Anaemia, leucocytosis and a raised ESR are common. At this stage, the serological tests are positive.

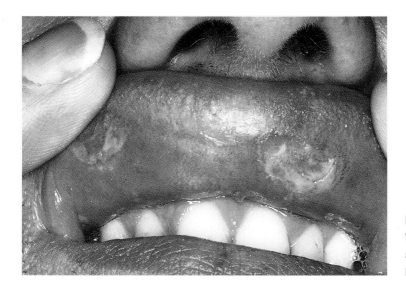

Fig. 1.60 Secondary syphilis. White, slightly eroded patches are present inside the upper lip. By courtesy of Dr. B. Monk.

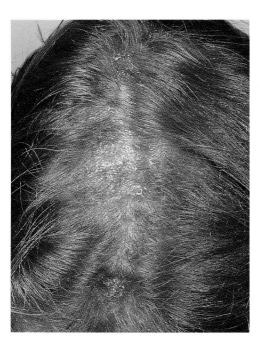

Fig. 1.61 Secondary syphilis. There are patches of erythema, scaling and alopecia in the scalp.

Secondary Relapse and Latent Syphilis

If untreated, the patient recovers with a variety of possible sequelae. There may be a secondary relapse of a mucocutaneous nature within two years. The eruption particularly affects the genitalia and palms and soles. This condition is still infectious. The disease then passes into a latent asymptomatic phase but with positive serology. Even during this phase, sero-negative conversion and spontaneous cure may occur. If it does not, the disease may proceed to cardiovascular or neurosyphilis or other organ involvement. This is known as tertiary syphilis.

Tertiary Syphilis

The gumma is the hallmark of tertiary syphilis. It is a chronic granuloma. It develops a number of years after the primary inoculation and is non-infectious. Only the mucocutaneous manifestations will be dealt with here.

The dermal gummata are firm brownish-red papules or nodules which are usually arranged in an annular pattern as raised plaques (Fig. 1.62). The lesions are asymmetrical and sparse or solitary, with a smooth, scaly surface, resembling psoriasis. They heal with scarring. Subcutaneous lesions may break down and ulcerate. The ulcer is several centimetres in diameter and has a vertical punched-out wall (Figs. 1.63 and 1.64). The base has a yellow slough rather like a chamois leather. These lesions occur particularly over the upper shins, the chest, face and scalp. Mucosal gummata may occur and the tongue may be diffusely infiltrated, producing white patches, erosions and fissuring. These may be premalignant.

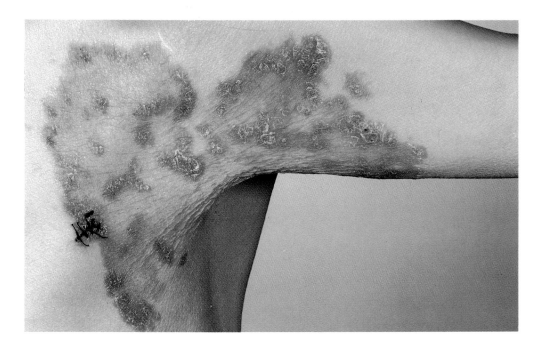

Fig. 1.62 Tertiary syphilis. The lesions are annular and consist of red-brown papules and infiltrated scaling plaques within the lesion. The diagnosis was suggested after a skin biopsy.

Congenital Syphilis

This disorder is extremely rare where routine ante-natal care demands serological examination of all expectant mothers. The result of transplacental infection depends on the immunological maturity of the fetus and the degree of the infection. Early in pregnancy, abortion or still-birth is the rule and the fetus is covered in blisters. If pregnancy progresses to a later stage, the child may be born with papules and blisters on the palms and soles, or born healthy with subsequent failure to thrive and an eruption similar to secondary syphilis with hepatosplenomegaly and pulmonary and bone involvement. Late congenital syphilis presents with tertiary-like manifestations in childhood. The stigmata include perforation of the palate and collapse of the nose due to gummata and frontal bossing and bowing of the tibia due to periostitis. Nerve deafness, abnormal teeth and interstitial keratitis (Hutchinson's triad) and joint effusions occur. Neurosyphilis may result.

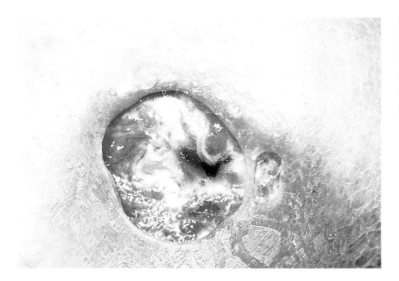

Fig. 1.63 Tertiary syphilis. The ulcer is well-defined with vertical edges and appears 'punched out'. The base has a yellow slough. By courtesy of St. Mary's Hospital.

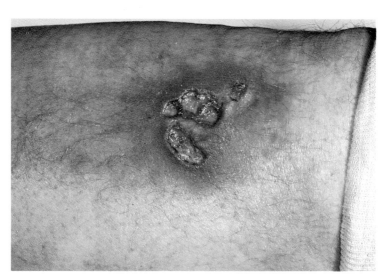

Fig. 1.64 Tertiary syphilis. The ulcers are well-defined with vertical edges. A skin biopsy is necessary to establish the diagnosis.

2

Viral Infections of the Skin

Many human viral disorders have cutaneous manifestations as part of a more general disturbance, for example measles and smallpox, but their description classically lies within the speciality of infectious diseases. The viral disorders which are referred to a dermatologist are described here and in the main they have little or no constitutional disturbance.

HERPES SIMPLEX

Herpes simplex is a double-stranded DNA virus which causes an acute self-limiting eruption on the skin or mucous membranes. When it occurs on the face, it is temporarily disfiguring but produces little morbidity. When it occurs on the genitalia, it can give rise to enormous distress and anxiety.

The disease is contagious and results in an initial primary infection (Figs. 2.1 and 2.2) which may be followed by recurrent attacks without further reinfection. During primary infection, the virus reaches the dorsal root ganglion via peripheral nerves, and it lies dormant there until it is subsequently reactivated. Primary infection often occurs in childhood and is acquired from a parent (Fig. 2.3); a gingivostomatitis may result. The severity of the infection varies but there is an incubation period of three to ten days followed by a fever and sore throat. Painful, grouped vesicles develop on the lips (Fig. 2.4), tongue, gums, buccal mucosae and palate. Erosion and crusting follow and regional lymphadenopathy is present. Primary infections may occur at other sites, particularly on the genitalia, in adults. Most individuals, however, have no personal or parental recollection of a primary infection and would appear to have had a subclinical primary infection as judged by the presence of antibodies and the tendency to recurrent attacks.

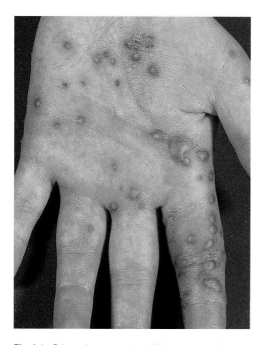
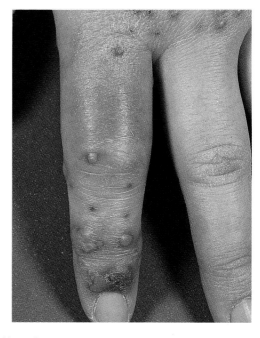

Fig. 2.1 Primary herpes simplex. Widespread vesicles surrounded by erythema are present on the back and front of the hand. Type II herpes simplex was recovered. By courtesy of Dr. Michèle Clement.

The herpes simplex virus is classified into Type I and Type II. Differentiation could originally be made on a clinical basis because Type II infections were limited to ano-genital sites, but this no longer pertains and laboratory tests are required to distinguish the two. Recurrent attacks occur within the area of the initial primary inoculation. The reason for recurrences may be obscure, but the most frequent causes are menstruation, sunlight, fever, stress, trauma and general illness. It is of note that lobar pneumonia is almost invariably accompanied by 'fever blisters', even in those who do not recall having had herpes simplex infections previously. The regularity of the recurrences varies greatly between individuals. Most have one or two a year but some seem to be rarely without attacks, especially in the case of genital lesions.

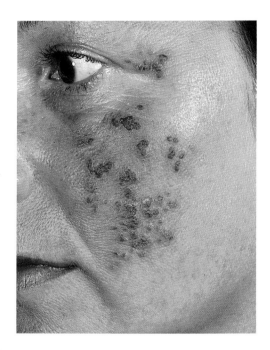

Fig. 2.2 Primary herpes simplex. Grouped crusted vesicles surrounded by erythema are present.

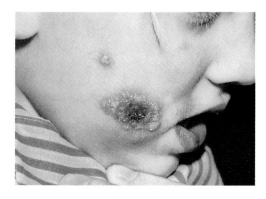

Fig. 2.3 Herpes simplex. The virus is often acquired when an infant or child is kissed by an infected parent. Grouped vesicles, crusting and erythema occur.

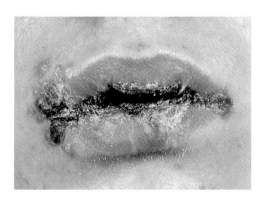

Fig. 2.4 Primary herpes simplex. A few vesicles are present but most of the lesions have become crusted. This was a primary attack of herpes simplex.

The eruption begins with tingling or discomfort in the skin and a cluster of lesions develops (Fig. 2.5). These evolve rapidly from a macule to a papule to a vesicle surrounded by erythema. The vesicles may coalesce. They dry and scab and, in the majority, heal without scarring. In some, however, they become eroded and necrotic and scarring may result. Secondary bacterial infection occasionally occurs (Fig. 2.6). The length of the attack varies from five to fourteen days.

Infection with herpes simplex may occur anywhere on the mucocutaneous surface but the commonest sites are the lips or face. The genital form (Fig. 2.7) has become increasingly frequent since the late 1960s. Part of the problem is that a woman may have an infection limited to the cervix and therefore experience no symptoms, so the disease is unwittingly transmitted. The virus is active during the vesicular stage and may be a hazard to medical and dental personnel. This may result in inoculation of the skin of an examining finger and result in a so-called 'herpetic whitlow' (Fig. 2.8).

In the main, the cold sore is an innocuous inconvenience but there are certain complications. The eye may become infected, with resultant keratitis and, occasionally, blindness. The early use of the anti-viral agents, has, however, been gratifyingly effective.

Sufferers from atopic eczema are particularly susceptible to the virus. The eczema becomes superimposed by the virus and a severe, potentially life-threatening illness known as 'eczema herpeticum' may result (Figs. 2.9 and 2.10). This, fortunately, now responds dramatically to the anti-viral agent acyclovir.

Herpes simplex infections are occasionally followed by erythema multiforme or Stevens–Johnson syndrome. The virus causes meningitis and encephalitis. The immunosuppressed are at risk, as are infants

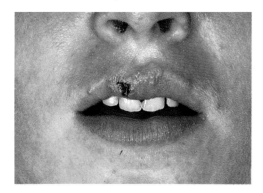

Fig. 2.5 Recurrent herpes simplex. The 'cold sore' occurs most commonly on the lips. Vesicles and crusting are present.

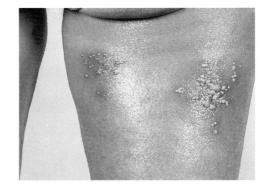

Fig. 2.6 Herpes simplex. The vesicles may become purulent with secondary bacterial infection.

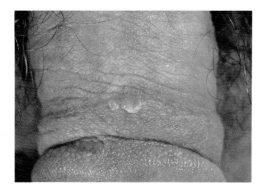

Fig. 2.7 Genital herpes simplex. This disorder is becoming common and causes considerable distress. By courtesy of St. John's Hospital for Diseases of the Skin.

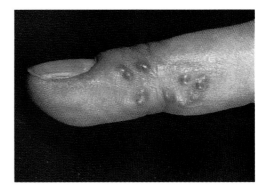

Fig. 2.8 Herpes simplex. Medical personnel and dentists may unwittingly contract the virus on a finger from tending an infected patient.

born to mothers with active herpes simplex cervicitis or vulvitis. This may result in disseminated cutaneous infection with severe neurological and other organ involvement. Maternal genital infection at the time of parturition is an indication for Caesarean section. Patients with advanced malignant disease, particularly those being treated with immunosuppressive drugs, are similarly at risk from the disseminated disease. There is evidence that the herpes simplex Type II virus could be implicated in the aetiology of carcinoma of the cervix. These women have a higher incidence of herpes simplex antibodies and the virus has been recovered from cell cultures of cervical carcinoma.

The specific treatment of viral disorders is still unsatisfactory. Undoubtedly, however, more progress has been made with the herpes simplex virus than most other viruses. Idoxuridine in dimethyl sulphoxide is being replaced by acyclovir. This drug reduces the length and the morbidity of recurrent attacks when applied topically, but does not prevent recurrences. Taken orally and continuously it does prevent recurrences. However, the attacks return on stopping the drug and the long-term hazards of continuous therapy are unknown. Oral and intravenous acyclovir have dramatically improved the treatment of eczema herpeticum and primary and disseminated infections.

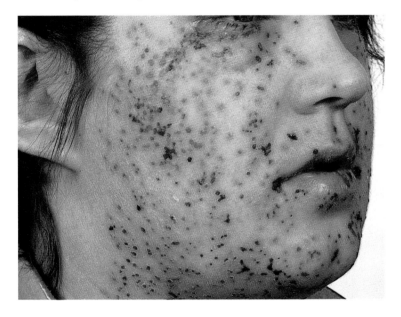

Fig. 2.9 Eczema herpeticum (Kaposi's varicelliform eruption). Eczematous subjects are prone to widespread herpes simplex infections.

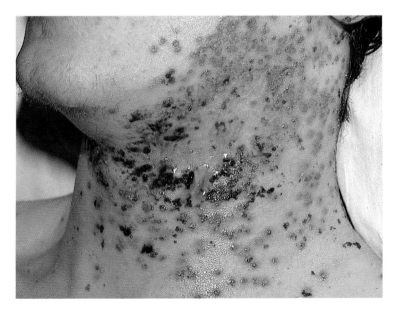

Fig. 2.10 Eczema herpeticum. A myriad of vesicles are present, surrounded by erythema with erosions centrally. Acyclovir has dramatically improved the treatment of this condition.

HERPES ZOSTER (Shingles)

Herpes zoster is an infection caused by the same virus as that which causes varicella (chickenpox) (Fig. 2.11). The disease represents a reactivation of the chickenpox virus which lies dormant in the dorsal root or cranial nerve ganglion after the initial attack. There may be an interval of several decades of latency before the virus spreads along the cutaneous nerves. Shingles cannot be caught from another individual; it occurs only in those carrying the dormant virus. The reactivation of the latent virus is a purely personal event. However, since live varicella virus is present in the lesions of shingles, chickenpox can be contracted by an individual who has never had chickenpox from a patient who is suffering from shingles.

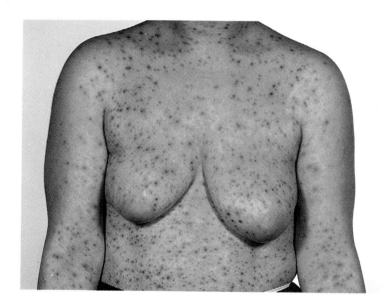

Fig. 2.11 Chickenpox (varicella). Chickenpox and shingles (herpes zoster) are caused by the same virus. Chickenpox may be contracted from a patient with herpes zoster but not vice-versa.

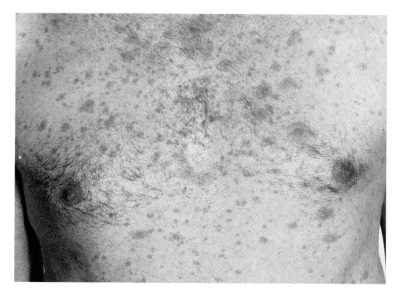

The first symptom is the fairly acute onset of pain or discomfort. By the time of presentation there is usually a vesicular eruption on one side of the body corresponding to a dermatome (Figs. 2.12–2.15).

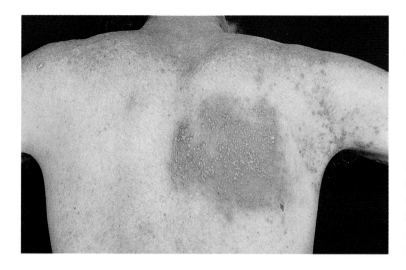

Fig. 2.12 Herpes zoster. The eruption occurs in a unilateral distribution, corresponding to the limits of a dermatome. By courtesy of St. John's Hospital for Diseases of the Skin.

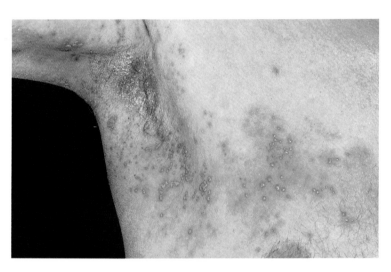

Fig. 2.13 Herpes zoster. Front view of the patient depicted in Fig. 2.12. By courtesy of St. John's Hospital for Diseases of the Skin.

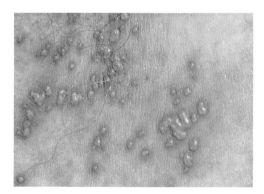

Fig. 2.14 Herpes zoster. Vesicles surrounded by erythema are the hallmark of shingles. This is a close-up of lesions in Fig. 2.13. By courtesy of St. John's Hospital for Diseases of the Skin.

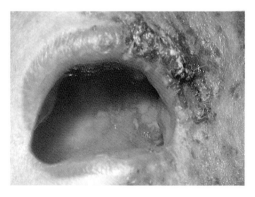

Fig. 2.15 Oral herpes zoster. Vesicles are present in the mucous membranes and on the skin in trigeminal nerve involvement. The eruption is unilateral. By courtesy of St. Mary's Hospital.

Each individual lesion commences as a macule which rapidly becomes a vesicle surrounded by erythema (Fig. 2.16). The lesions evolve over the next two or three weeks, becoming pustular, haemorrhagic (Fig. 2.17) and finally scabbed (Fig. 2.18). As the scabs fall off, a scar may result (Fig. 2.19). The lesions are to be found at various stages of development. Many become confluent. There are usually satellite lesions to be found elsewhere on the body away from the originally involved dermatome. Secondary bacterial sepsis is common. There may be associated local lymphadenopathy.

For most individuals, an attack of shingles represents a tiresome interlude of two to three weeks during which they feel unwell and uncomfortable but make a full recovery with no sequelae. However, involvement of certain dermatomes may have important complications. Thus, the eye may be involved (Fig. 2.20) if the ophthalmic branch of the trigeminal nerve is attacked. This requires urgent treatment with acyclovir to prevent permanent damage. In these cases, the ciliary ganglion is usually involved and there are vesicles on the side and the tip of the nose. Involvement of the geniculate ganglion gives rise to Ramsay Hunt's syndrome. This is a facial nerve palsy with involvement of the external ear, or tympanic membrane. There may be tinnitis, vertigo and deafness. Involvement of the sacral nerves may be extremely debilitating and may lead to difficulties with micturition and defaecation. Paralysis of an upper or lower limb (usually temporary) may occur secondary to disruption of motor nerves involved by the dermatome. The elderly are particularly at risk from herpes zoster, for there is a significant incidence of post-herpetic neuralgia which may be intractable and very disheartening.

The factors governing the reactivation of the dormant chickenpox virus are unknown, but clearly, immunosuppressed individuals are at risk. Patients with lymphoma, particularly those undergoing

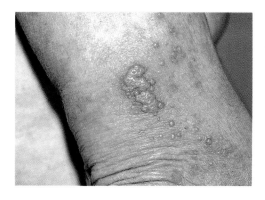

Fig. 2.16 Herpes zoster. Vesicles are surrounded by erythema and subsequently become confluent.

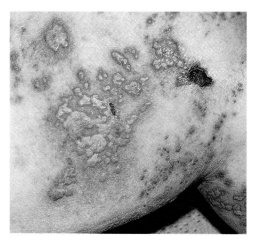

Fig. 2.17 Herpes zoster. The lesions become more haemorrhagic and turbid as they progress.

Fig. 2.18 Satellite zoster. Satellite vesicles are usually found away from the involved dermatome in most patients.

therapy with immunosuppressive drugs, may develop widespread disease such that in addition to the initial single dermatome involvement, there are lesions all over the cutaneous surface, as in chickenpox (Fig. 2.21). In such individuals, the disorder may be life-threatening with visceral, pulmonary hepatic and neurological involvement.

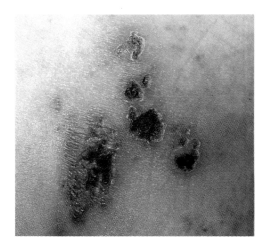

Fig. 2.19 Herpes zoster. Necrotic lesions result and scarring is common following the disorder. By courtesy of St. Mary's Hospital.

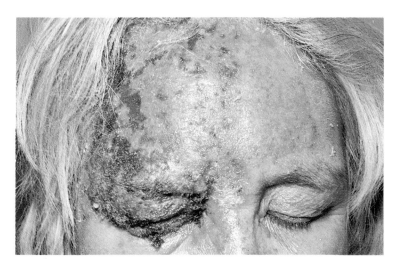

Fig. 2.20 Ophthalmic zoster. Crusting and erosion are present. The ophthalmic branch of the right trigeminal nerve is affected. It is essential to treat the eye if it is involved. By courtesy of St. Mary's Hospital.

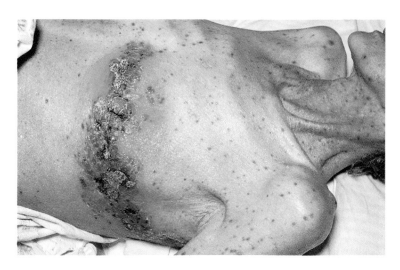

Fig. 2.21 Disseminated zoster. In the immunosuppressed, the virus may be disseminated to involve most of the cutaneous surface as in chickenpox. By courtesy of St. Bartholomew's Hospital.

Treatment is still unsatisfactory. For the majority, adequate analgesia is enough. Some authorities have advocated high doses of systemic steroids as anti-inflammatory agents in an attempt to prevent post-herpetic neuralgia in the elderly. Forty percent idoxuridine in DMSO has been used topically with some degree of success. Systemic acyclovir is now the treatment of choice for herpes zoster in the immunosuppressed.

VACCINIA

Vaccination against smallpox with the vaccinia virus is no longer routine since the virtual eradication of the disease worldwide, so complications of the technique are no longer likely to be encountered. Bacterial sepsis of the vaccination site is the most common complication, but toxic eruptions such as erythema multiforme may also occur. *In utero*, in infants, in the immunosuppressed and in eczema, generalized or progressive vaccinia may occur. Encephalitis is a rare complication. Accidental autoinoculation from the vaccination site occasionally results in an eruption of umbilicated vesicles identical to those of the initial vaccination (Fig. 2.22).

WARTS

These are an extremely common, self-limiting condition of the skin or mucous membranes, particularly in the young. The causative papilloma virus can infect many sites and is serologically different in each area. Warts are harmless but give rise to symptoms because they are unsightly, embarrassing and painful, particularly on the feet. They are infectious and may be contracted from other individuals or from swimming pools and public changing facilities.

Common Warts

Common warts are seen most often on the hands and fingers (Fig. 2.23) and around the nails. However, they may occur anywhere on the body. Clinically, they are firm, discrete papules with a rough, 'warty' surface. They vary in size from one millimetre to well over a centimetre. They may be single or multiple, and occasionally they coalesce and may produce larger masses.

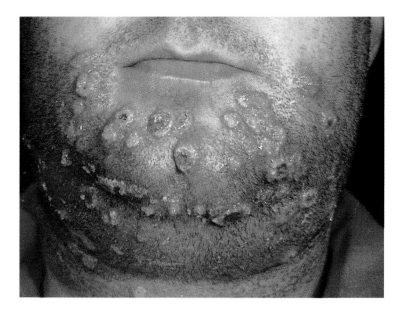

Fig. 2.22 Vaccinia. Accidental autoinoculation of the virus from a vaccination site results in umbilicated vesicles identical to those of the original vaccination.

Plane Warts

Plane warts are very small lesions which are just slightly raised with a smooth, flat, skin-coloured or slightly pigmented surface (Figs. 2.24 and 2.25). They occur particularly on the face and the backs of the hands. They are often misdiagnosed, probably because they are quite small and do not have a rough, 'warty' surface and are erroneously treated with topical glucocorticosteroids, in which case they spread. Frequently, they occur in lines corresponding to a scratch or some other such trauma. This is known as the Koebner phenomenon. Plane warts may be peculiarly persistent.

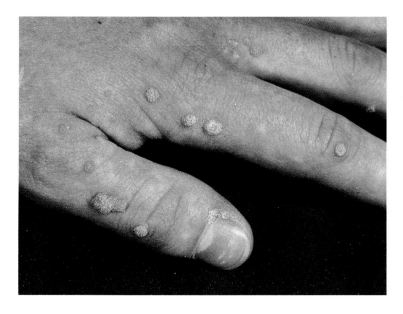

Fig. 2.23 Common warts. The hands and fingers are the most common sites. The lesions are discrete, firm papules with a rough surface.

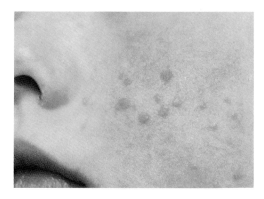

Fig. 2.24 Plane warts. Discrete slightly raised small lesions occur on the face. They are often mistaken for acne or, worse, for eczema and mistreated with topical steroids, in which case they spread.

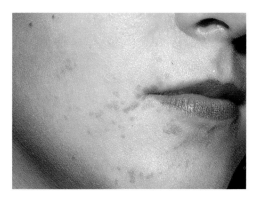

Fig. 2.25 Plane warts. The lesions may be quite pigmented. They are often persistent.

Plantar Warts

Plantar warts are often known colloquially as 'verrucae'. Single lesions may occur but frequently they coalesce and then are known as 'mosaic' warts (Fig. 2.26). If they occur on the direct pressure-bearing areas of the feet they can be painful and interfere with walking. Because direct pressure forces them deep into the dermis they are flat, almost circular lesions, with a rough surface. Pin-point black spots may be seen on the surface due to thrombosed capillaries. The capillaries will bleed on paring the wart and serve to differentiate them from corns (callosities). A corn (Figs. 2.27 and 2.28) represents a thickening of the skin overlying a bony prominence, resulting from friction between the skin, the bony prominence and tight-fitting shoes. The skin becomes more and more normal looking on paring in contrast to a wart. Plantar warts can be extremely persistent.

Filiform or Digitate Warts

Filiform or digitate warts are often found on the face, neck or anogenital area (Figs. 2.29–2.32). In the latter site they are known as 'condylomata accuminata'. They may invade the vagina, urethra or rectum. Certain serological types may be implicated in cervical carcinoma.

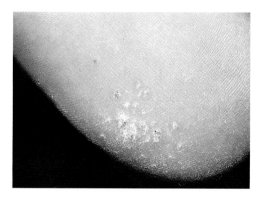

Fig. 2.26 Plantar warts (verrucae). The lesions are frequently multiple and coalesce to produce a mosaic pattern. They are well-defined and have a rough surface. They bleed on paring.

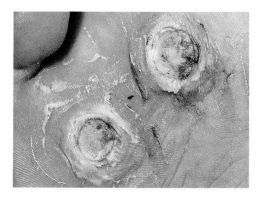

Fig. 2.27 Corns. A corn is a thickening of the skin resulting from friction. On the sole they occur over bony prominences and are distinguished from verrucae because the skin appears more normal on paring and does not bleed.

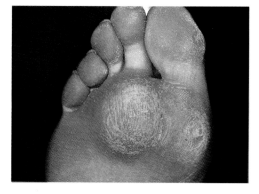

Fig. 2.28 Callosities. The hyperkeratotic skin has occurred over the metatarsal phalangeal joints and the medial side of the big toe, areas which are easily compressed by ill-fitting shoes.

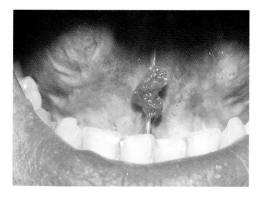

Fig 2.29 Digitate (filiform) warts. Warts may occur on mucous membanes. This wart was probably contracted sexually.

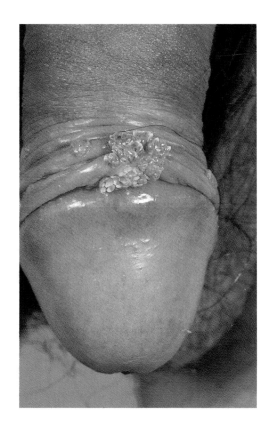

Fig. 2.30 Penile warts. Filiform warts on the genitalia are usually sexually transmitted and the patient should be screened for other sexually transmissible disorders.

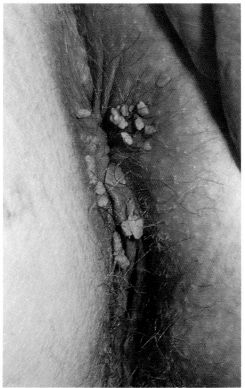

Fig. 2.31 Perianal warts. Discrete raised pedunculated warty lesions are present. They may be treated with podophyllin applied by an experienced operator (or else a perilesional dermatitis may occur), liquid nitrogen or surgery.

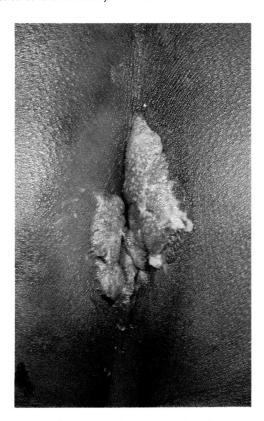

Fig. 2.32 Perianal warts. Large accumulations of warts may occur especially if they are initially treated with topical steroids. The source of these warts in this ten-year-old was not established.

The treatment of warts is unsatisfactory. There are no suitable anti-viral agents available. All warts ultimately resolve so that conservative measures are usually preferred, especially since recurrences are common. Salycilic acid, podophyllin and formalin are the mainstays of conservative therapy. Applications of liquid nitrogen are effective for warts in most sites but may be painful, especially on the feet. Surgery is useful for single lesions.

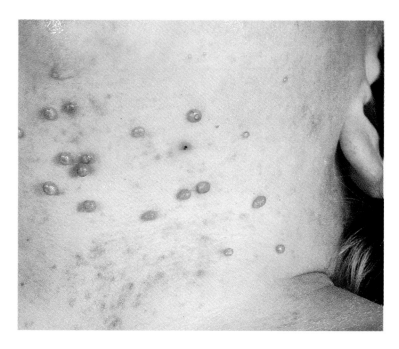

Fig. 2.33 Molluscum contagiosum. Several discrete dome-shaped papules are present on the neck of this two-year-old.

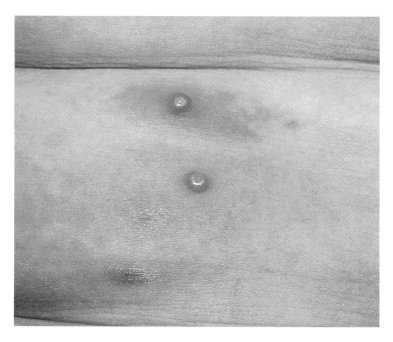

Fig. 2.34 Molluscum contagiosum. A central depression ('umbilication') is visible on the surface of the lesions.

MOLLUSCUM CONTAGIOSUM

This is a common eruption affecting the skin and mucous membranes and is caused by a large DNA virus which is a member of the pox group. The lesions are flesh-coloured, dome-shaped papules (Fig. 2.33) which vary in size from minute lesions to a centimetre or so in diameter. A central depression is visible in the surface of the lesion (Fig. 2.34). This 'umbilication' is a most important diagnostic sign. The lesions occur anywhere on the body but particularly on the face and trunk in children and around the genitalia in adults (Fig. 2.35). The lesions are fairly infectious. Children acquire them from one another at school, and swimming pools are common sources of infection. Genital lesions in adults (Fig. 2.36) are usually acquired sexually. The lesions disappear spontaneously after several months.

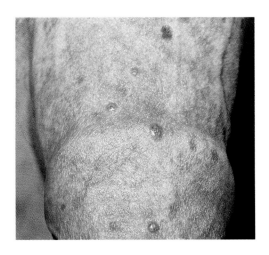

Fig. 2.35 Genital molluscum contagiosum. These lesions are contracted sexually.

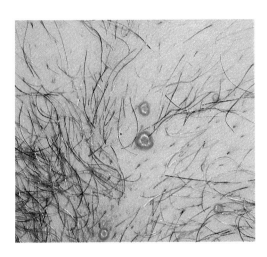

Fig. 2.36 Pubic molluscum contagiosum. It is wise to screen for other sexually transmissable diseases in adults with genital lesions.

As they disappear they often develop a surrounding patch of eczema (Fig. 2.37). They can vary in number from a single lesion (Figs. 2.38 and 2.39), which may be difficult to diagnose prior to histological examination, to multiple lesions. Patients with eczema are prone to this infection. The lesions are then commonly mistaken for the eczema and are inappropriately treated with topical steroids and therefore spread extensively. The lesions respond well to treatment by destructive methods such as liquid nitrogen therapy, curettage and cautery, or piercing the lesions with an orange-stick dipped in aqueous phenol or iodine. Once they have gone they rarely recur.

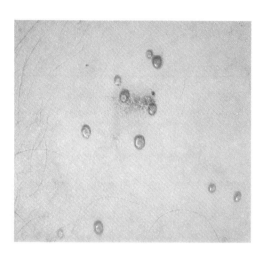

Fig. 2.37 Molluscum contagiosum. Eczema frequently develops around the lesions as they resolve.

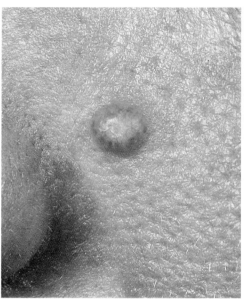

Fig. 2.38 Solitary molluscum contagiosum. The central depression in the surface of the lesion is a helpful diagnostic physical sign.

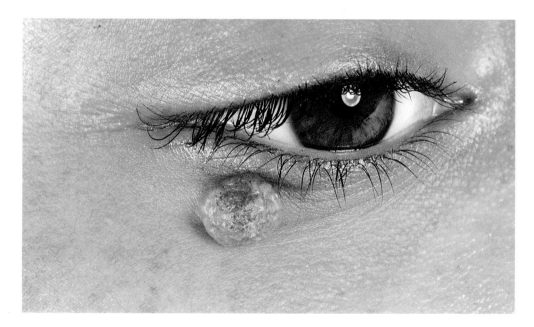

Fig. 2.39 Solitary molluscum contagiosum. Solitary lesions may be difficult to diagnose clinically. They are often quite large ('giant molluscum'). This lesion is well-defined, raised and dome-shaped and there is central change.

ORF

This condition is also due to a pox virus and is contracted from infected sheep. The condition causes vesicles around the mouth of the animals and is sometimes known as 'scabby mouth'. The virus survives on fences and feeding troughs from which the infection may be acquired. The disease occurs in butchers (Fig. 2.40), meat porters and farmers and others who have occasion to encounter contaminated material.

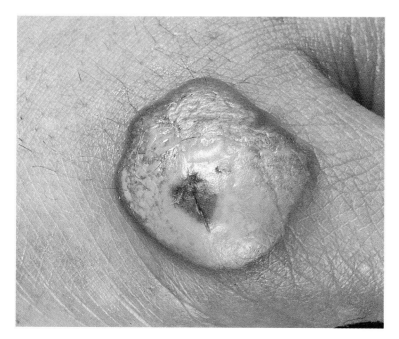

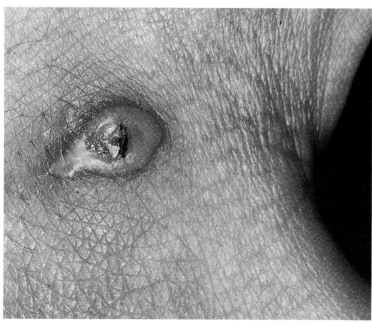

Fig. 2.40 Orf. The lesion is vesicular and weeps. These two Arab brothers were amateur butchers preparing halal meat for Ramadan. They had not recognized the sheep's 'scabby mouth'.

There is usually a solitary lesion on a finger, which lasts just over a month. It is a papule with the characteristic appearance of a red centre surrounded by a white ring, with red in the periphery (Figs. 2.41 and 2.42). It weeps and then crusts over before separating away from the underlying healing skin. There is frequently regional lymphadenopathy and a fever. Occasionally, a toxic eruption, such as erythema multiforme, occurs in addition. There is no specific treatment.

HAND, FOOT AND MOUTH DISEASE

This is a disorder of children and young adults. It is caused by a Coxsackievirus, usually of the A16 strain. This is an enterovirus of the picorna family. There is a three-day incubation period during which the virus enters via the buccal mucosa and the small intestine. It travels to the regional lymph nodes and

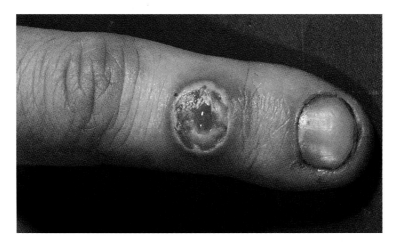

Fig. 2.41 Orf. The lesion often has a red centre, surrounded by white with red at the periphery.

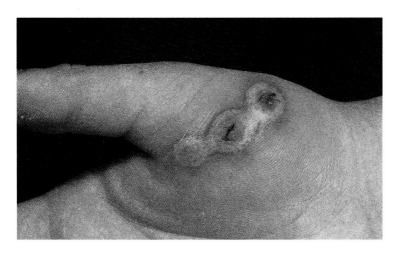

Fig. 2.42 Orf. The fingers or hand are the most common sites. It is contracted from sheep infected with the virus. Three lesions are present.

there is then a generalized viraemia with localizing of the virus to the mouth, hands and feet. The condition lasts about seven days. The clinical picture is distinctive. There are a limited number of oval, slightly yellow, vesicles surrounded by erythema on the hands and feet (Fig. 2.43). In the mouth, erosions (Fig. 2.44) are more common since the roof of the vesicle is quickly removed by the tongue. There is a mild systemic disturbance and the condition does not usually recur.

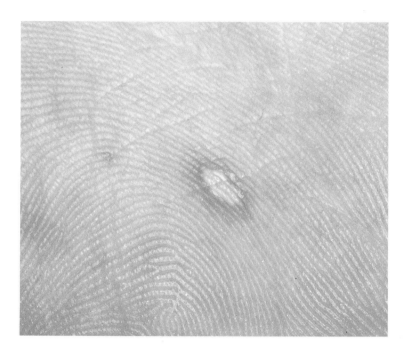

Fig. 2.43 Hand, foot and mouth disease. The lesion is an oval white vesicle surrounded by erythema on the palm. There are usually only a few lesions. By courtesy of St. Bartholomew's Hospital.

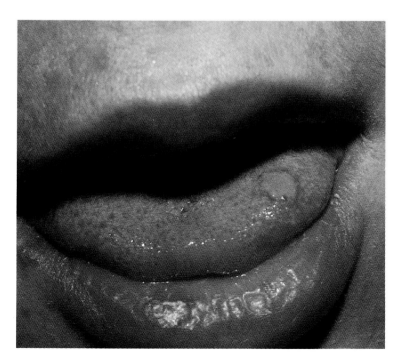

Fig. 2.44 Hand, foot and mouth disease. Discrete, small oval or round erosions occur in the mouth. The disorder is self-limiting and caused by Coxsackievirus.

3

Fungal Infections of the Skin

Superficial fungal disorders of the skin are very common and usually respond admirably to treatment. If misdiagnosed, however, they are almost invariably treated with topical glucocorticosteroids and since these drugs are immunosuppressives, the fungi will flourish and the disease process worsen.

PITYRIASIS VERSICOLOR

This is a common, insidious condition of young, healthy adults caused by *Pityrosporum orbiculare*, a lipophilic yeast. It occurs after puberty and the development of mature sebaceous glands. The yeast is a unicellular commensal of normal skin but in the pathogenic state it reproduces by budding and produces filaments known as pseudohyphae. In this form the organism is known as *Malassezia furfur*. The yeast is an opportunist. Pathogenicity is encouraged by an increase in environmental temperature and humidity, such that many individuals notice its presence after a summer vacation. It is also a common cutaneous complication in individuals who are immunosuppressed, either through disease, for example lymphoma, or through drugs, for example systemic steroids.

The physical signs are small macules which coalesce as they increase in size, so that lesions of various shapes and sizes occur (Fig. 3.1). They tend to surround the orifices of hair follicles. The fungus is keratinophilic and thus occurs in the stratum corneum and produces scaling (Fig. 3.2). This scaling may not be immediately obvious on examination but can be demonstrated by gentle scraping of a lesion with a blunt scalpel. The colour of the lesions varies (hence 'versicolor') but is distinctive. In the pale, non-suntanned Caucasian the lesions are brown or fawn-coloured (Fig. 3.3). In the suntanned individual the lesions appear pale in comparison with the surrounding normal skin (Fig. 3.4). This was originally thought to be caused by the fungus shielding the melanocytes from ultra-violet light irradiation. However, it is now clear that dicarboxylic acids produced by the fungus temporarily impair melanocytic function and thus cause hypopigmentation. In any one individual, including dark-skinned people, both hyper- (Fig. 3.5) and hypopigmented lesions (Fig. 3.6) may occur.

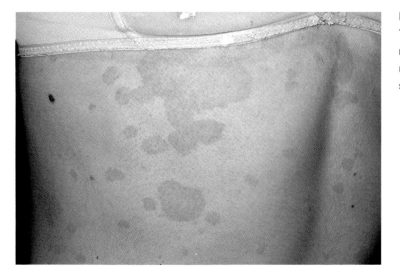

Fig. 3.1 Pityriasis versicolor. The lesions commence as small macules which coalesce resulting in lesions of different shapes and sizes.

The eruption is asymmetrical and occurs on the back, chest (Fig. 3.7) and neck. It is most unusual to see the disease on the face, despite the fact that it is well supplied by sebaceous glands. The explanation for this is not clear, but possibly covered areas of the body produce the occlusive environment which favours pathogenicity. In widespread cases, especially those mistreated with topical steroids (Fig. 3.8), lesions may also occur on the limbs.

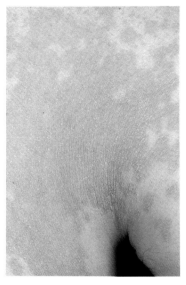

Fig. 3.2 Pityriasis versicolor. Slight scaling is just visible. Gentle scraping of the lesions with a blunt scalpel will enhance the scaling.

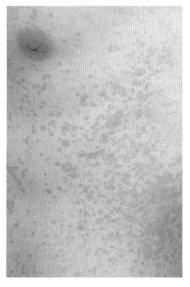

Fig. 3.3 Pityriasis versicolor. Fawn-coloured or brown macules coalesce to produce confluent patches.

Fig. 3.4 Pityriasis versicolor. The fungus produces dicarboxylic acids which temporarily impair melanocytic function resulting in hypopigmented macules.

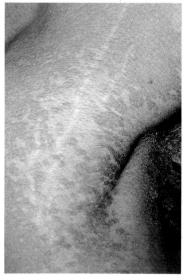

Fig. 3.5 Pityriasis versicolor. Hyperpigmented macules are present in this West Indian.

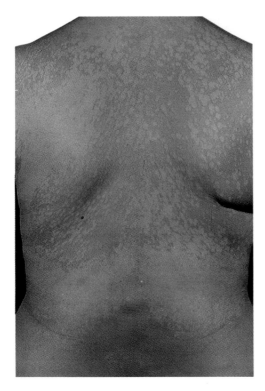

Fig. 3.6 Pityriasis versicolor. Both hypo- and hyperpigmented lesions may occur in one individual.

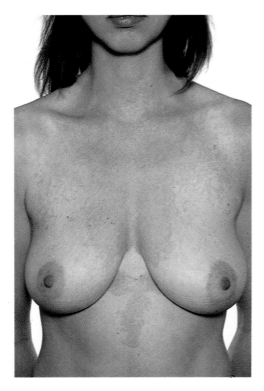

Fig. 3.7 Pityriasis versicolor. The eruption occurs mainly on the torso.

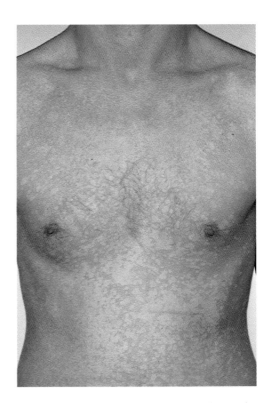

Fig. 3.8 Pityriasis versicolor. Hypo- and hyperpigmented macules are present. The eruption becomes widespread if mistreated with topical steroids.

The diagnosis can be confirmed by taking scrapings of the skin with a blunt scalpel. The scales are put on a microscope slide and 30% potassium hydroxide solution is added. The thick-walled, spherical yeasts with pseudohyphae may then be seen. Certain ink stains are taken up by the organism, giving a better microscopic preparation (Fig. 3.9). This fungus is not readily grown on culture media and therefore culture methods are not routinely performed.

The fungus is easily treated. Half-strength Whitfield's ointment, selenium sulphide shampoo or topical applications of imidazoles are all effective. Systemic ketoconazole, 200mg daily for five days, is also curative but should only be used rarely because it is a potentially hepatotoxic agent. The condition often recurs either because of inadequate therapy or because of a resurgence of the original precipitating factors. It should be noted that pityriasis versicolor does not respond to oral griseofulvin unlike tinea infections. In order to avoid confusion, the condition's alternative name, tinea versicolor, is better abandoned.

Complete resolution of the rash occurs within three or four weeks of treatment. However, in those who have pronounced hypopigmentation, although the scaling (the sign of active pityriasis versicolor) disappears, white areas remain (Fig. 3.10) simulating vitiligo. It is usually several months before the melanocytes recover and start producing pigment again.

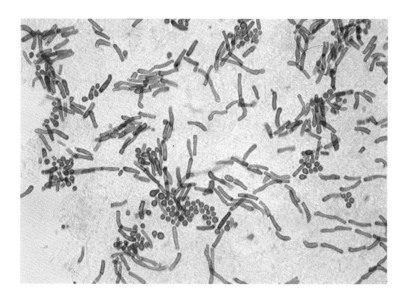

Fig. 3.9 Pityriasis versicolor. *Malassezia furfur* is found in the skin. Parker's stain (equal parts 30% potassium hydroxide and Parker's blue-black ink) (× 128). By courtesy of Miss G. Midgley, St. John's Hospital for Diseases of the Skin.

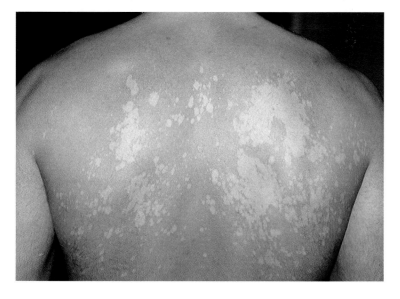

Fig. 3.10 Pityriasis versicolor. The hypopigmentation may be mistaken for vitiligo, especially after treatment, but the lesions are asymmetrical, of various shapes and sizes and confined to the torso unlike vitiligo.

CANDIDA ALBICANS

Candida albicans is a yeast (Figs. 3.11 and 3.12). It is a commensal of the gastrointestinal, upper respiratory and genital tracts and also of warm and moist skinfolds. It becomes pathogenic quite readily and particularly favours a warm, occluded, wet environment. The disease states that result are oral and genital candidosis (mucous membrane candidosis, commonly known as thrush), candida intertrigo and chronic paronychia.

Oral Candidosis

Certain groups of individuals are at risk. The condition is common in infancy where immunological defence mechanisms are poorly-developed and the infection is frequently contracted from the genital tract of the mother. Ill and debilitated patients are particularly susceptible. These patients are usually immunosuppressed, either because of their underlying condition or because they are being treated with immunosuppressive drugs (particularly systemic steroids). Alternatively, broad spectrum antibiotics alter the normal bacterial flora permitting *Candida* to take their place. Otherwise healthy individuals who are edentulous, wear dentures and have poor dental hygiene are at risk. The denture provides occlusion which in turn implies increased moisture and warmth: the ideal environmental conditions for the overgrowth of *Candida albicans*.

The diagnosis of oral candidosis is not difficult. Well-defined white or yellow pustules (Fig. 3.13) or plaques are visible on the palate, tongue, buccal mucous membranes or gums. The lesions are easily scraped away with a spatula leaving a red, raw, bleeding base.

The condition responds to treatment of the predisposing conditions and the use of nystatin or one of the imidazoles. Oral ketoconazole is also effective but rarely required.

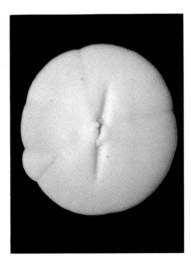

Fig. 3.11 *Candida albicans. Candida albicans* is a yeast. It has a pasty appearance on culture. By courtesy of Dr. Y.M. Clayton, St. John's Hospital for Diseases of the Skin.

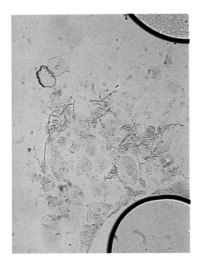

Fig. 3.12 Candida albicans. Candida albicans in 30% potassium hydroxide (× 128). By courtesy of Miss G. Midgley, St. John's Hospital for Diseases of the Skin.

Angular Cheilitis (Perlèche)

Although a disorder classically associated with the undernourished, this is most commonly seen in patients who wear dentures which do not fit properly. The conformation of the mouth becomes distorted and sags, such that the upper lip tends to overhang the lower and a groove is formed at the angles of the mouth (Fig. 3.14). Saliva trickles imperceptibly down the fold providing a perfect habitat for *Candida albicans* to flourish. The area is sore, red, scaling and often fissured. Swabs taken from the cheilitis will confirm the condition. Sometimes, *Staphylococcus aureus* colonizes the area in addition to *Candida* or it may occur on its own. Swabs from the denture and mouth may also be positive for *Candida*. The condition responds to correcting the dentures and also to improvement in oral hygiene. It is important that the patients do not sleep in their dentures and are also taught to sterilize the dentures properly.

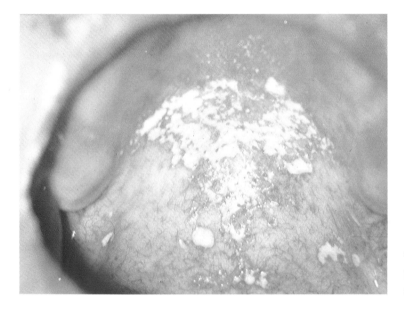

Fig. 3.13 Oral candidosis. White and yellow pustules are present on the palate. By courtesy of St. Mary's Hospital.

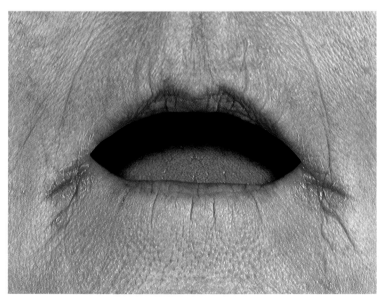

Fig. 3.14 Angular cheilitis. The condition occurs in the edentulous, especially those whose dentures are ill-fitting such that the conformation of the mouth is altered.

Candida Vulvo-vaginitis

Candida vaginitis is very common in young women. It may be precipitated by oral contraceptive therapy, pregnancy or systemic broad-spectrum antibiotics, all of which may alter the local flora. Fashionable, tight-fitting clothing produces an occluded, warm and moist environment which exacerbates the problem. Severe pruritus and soreness result, with a thick, abundant cream-coloured discharge. There is associated erythema and oedema. This is a common presentation of diabetes mellitus in middle-aged, often overweight women and it is mandatory to test the urine of any female presenting

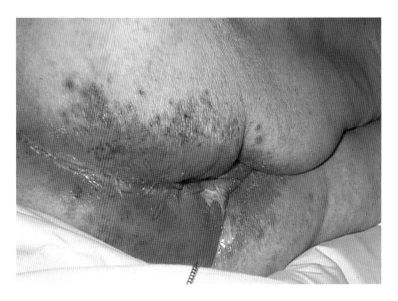

Fig. 3.15 Perineal candidosis. The skin becomes red and raw with discrete satellite pustules.

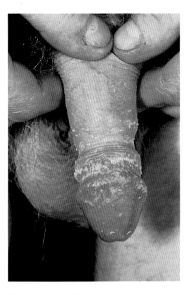

Fig. 3.16 Candida balanitis. The glans is studded with yellow pustules. It is more common in the uncircumcized. By courtesy of Dr. F. Lim.

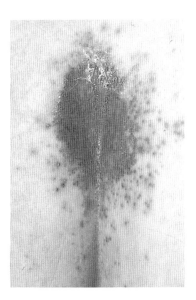

Fig. 3.17 Candida intertrigo. A raw erythema is present in the natal cleft with satellite pustules away from the central eruption. This lady was found to have glycosuria.

with candida vaginitis. If the vaginitis is neglected, the adjoining skin becomes involved. The appearances are of red, raw, glazed, oedematous skin (Fig. 3.15). The margin of the eruption is macerated and pustules seen away from the main body of the eruption are typical.

Predisposing causes should be attended to and the condition is treated with nystatin or imidazole pessaries. Recurrent attacks may be particularly troublesome. It may be necessary to sterilize the bowel with oral nystatin and occasionally, specific oral anti-candida treatment such as ketoconazole is necessary.

Candida Balanitis

Balanitis is usually contracted from a sexual partner with active disease. It is much more common in the uncircumcized since the prepuce provides an ideal occluded environment for the yeast to flourish. The glans may be red and swollen and studded with yellow pustules (Fig. 3.16). The condition responds to topical anti-candida agents.

Candida Intertrigo

Intertrigo is a dermatological term used to indicate a skin eruption occurring in an area between two opposing surfaces of the skin (Fig. 3.17). The axillae (Fig. 3.18), the groin (Fig. 3.19) and under the breasts are the major intertriginous areas. However, the interdigital, umbilical and other folds (particularly those occurring in the obese) and the posterior nailfolds are also intertriginous sites. There are various skin diseases which have a predilection for these areas, which include psoriasis, seborrhoeic eczema, erythrasma and tinea. An intertriginous site is ideal for candidosis because it is warm, moist and subject to friction and thus damage to the stratum corneum. Occlusive dressings or clothing, including napkins in infants, compound the problem.

The initial lesions are pustules on an erythematous base which become confluent. These break leaving red and raw skin. The outer margins of the eruption are often macerated. Maceration is a term used to describe excessive hydration of the stratum corneum. The skin appears thickened, white and sodden. Satellite lesions are characteristic and consist of fresh pustules away from the central core of the rash.

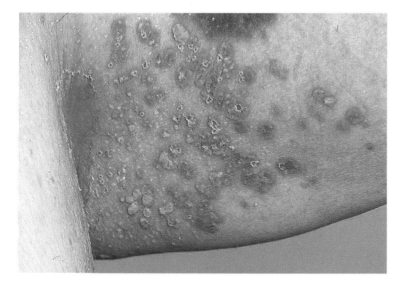

Fig. 3.18 Candida intertrigo. This lady had injured her arm in a fall; the bruising is evident. An eruption occurred between the two apposing skin surfaces because she was unwilling to move the arm. An erythema is present in the axilla and pustules are radiating out from it. By courtesy of St. Mary's Hospital.

Erosio Interdigitale

The apposing folds of skin between the fingers are not usually colonized by *Candida* but if the skin becomes damp and macerated because of too much immersion in water it becomes an ideal environment. There is a central red, raw and eroded area surrounded by maceration of the skin (Figs. 3.20 and 3.21).

Chronic Mucocutaneous Candidosis

This is an extremely rare disorder. A detailed description is not appropriate here, suffice to say that chronic mucocutaneous changes occur as a result of various immunological defects, particulary of cell-mediated immunity, in association with multiple endocrine defects or thymoma. Their delineation is the province of the immunologist but the clinical features are those of persistent oral thrush, often producing

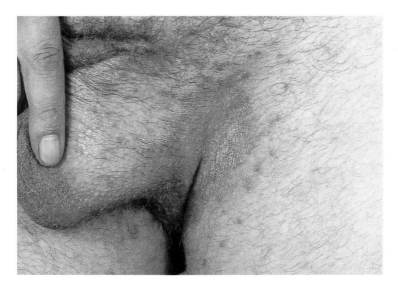

Fig. 3.19 Candida intertrigo. There is maceration in the fold with satellite pustules on the thighs and scrotum.

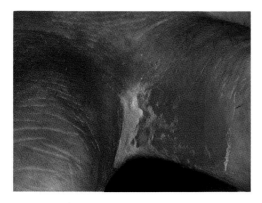

Fig. 3.20 Erosio interdigitale. There is maceration and erosion in the web between the fingers. This woman was a domestic and always had her hands in and out of water. Wet, occluded skin is ideal for colonization by *Candida albicans*.

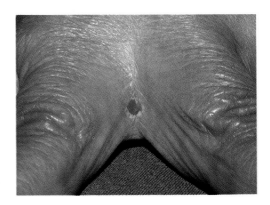

Fig. 3.21 Erosio interdigitale. This is a very early lesion. There is a central erosion surrounded by maceration. This occurred in a gynaecologist who was continually washing her hands after each consultation but not drying them carefully enough.

chronic hypertrophic changes, vulvo-vaginitis and destructive nail changes from chronic paronychia (Fig. 3.22). There are often widespread cutaneous hypertrophic plaques over the face, hands and elsewhere. Advances in immunotherapy and the availability of ketoconazole have vastly improved the treatment of this distressing condition.

TINEA (Ringworm)

Ringworm is a superficial fungal disorder of the skin. The fungus lives in dead keratin, that is, in the hair, nails or stratum corneum. It does not, ordinarily, penetrate deeper into the living cells. The fungus is a dermatophyte, a multicellular organism characterized by hyphae, which mat together to form mycelia. The hyphae can be seen on direct microscopy of the affected hair, nails or skin scales treated with potassium hydroxide (Fig. 3.23). The dermatophytes reproduce by spore formation. Vegetative arthrospores may be visible on direct microscopy but asexual spores are only produced after culture of material on Sabouraud's medium. This takes about three weeks. The asexual spores are known as macroconidia. There are three genera of dermatophytes which are identified by their macroconidia. They are known as *Microsporum*, *Epidermophyton* and *Trichophyton*. Thus, the individual genus and its species cannot be identified prior to culture but certain clinical characteristics of the infection may suggest the presence of one dermatophyte rather than another.

Ringworm infections may be described under their causative genera but it is customary to describe the infections in relation to their site on the skin.

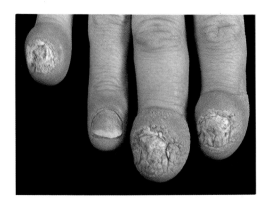

Fig. 3.22 Chronic mucocutaneous candidosis. Persistent nailfold erythema and oedema and severe dystrophic changes in the nails occur as a result of colonization by *Candida* due to immunoparesis. By courtesy of St. John's Hospital for Diseases of the Skin.

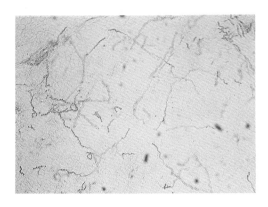

Fig. 3.23 Dermatophyte hyphae. Hyphae are present in scrapings of skin treated with potassium hydroxide (× 32). By courtesy of Miss G. Midgley, St. John's Hospital for Diseases of the Skin.

Ringworm of the scalp presents as one or several patches of hair loss coupled with various degrees of inflammation of the skin. There may, in addition, be lesions elsewhere. The pattern of hair loss depends on the amount of damage done by the fungus. Certain fungi invade the outer root sheath of the hair (ectothrix, Fig. 3.24). The affected hairs are broken off above the surface of the scalp and the coating of spores gives the hair a rather dull appearance. Other fungi invade the inner hair shaft itself (endothrix, Fig. 3.25). The damage done by the hyphae and the spores is considerable such that the hairs are broken off close to the surface. The inflammatory changes depend on whether the fungus is of human (anthropophilic) or animal (zoophilic) origin. With a human ringworm infection, the inflammatory changes may be quite minor (Fig. 3.26) but with an animal infection, host resistance is high and considerable inflammation (Fig. 3.27) may result in a boggy mass known as kerion. The patterns of tinea capitis are traditionally typed into ectothrix and endothrix infections, kerion and a fourth category known as favus.

Ectothrix Infections

SMALL-SPORED ECTOTHRIX FUNGI. These all belong to the *Microsporum* genus. They are the most common ringworm infections of the scalp. They are virtually never seen after puberty, probably because growth is inhibited by fatty acids produced by the mature sebaceous glands. Thus, a child with the disorder would

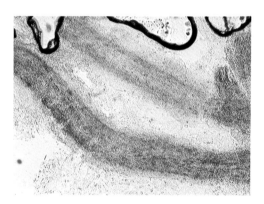

Fig. 3.24 Small-spored ectothrix. Infection of the outer hair root sheath is caused by *Microsporum* species. 30% potassium hydroxide preparation ($\times$ 32). By courtesy of Miss G. Midgley, St. John's Hospital for Diseases of the Skin.

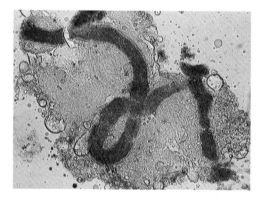

Fig. 3.25 Endothrix infection. The fungus invades the inner hair shaft. 30% potassium hydroxide preparation ($\times$ 96). By courtesy of Miss G. Midgley.

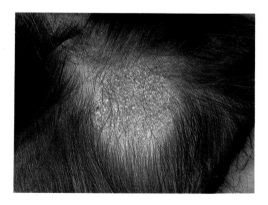

Fig. 3.26 Tinea capitis. In anthropophilic infections there is minimal scaling with loss of hair.

recover spontaneously at puberty. There are two common species – *M. canis.* (Fig. 3.28) and *M. audouinii.* The former is zoophilic (originating in either a cat or dog) and the latter is anthropophilic. The fungi invade the outer hair shaft and deposit their spores. These spores can be seen on direct microscopy. Hairs infected with either of these fungi fluoresce a brilliant green colour (Fig. 3.29) under an ultra-violet lamp emitting radiation at 360nm (Wood's light). Infections with human ringworm are highly contagious and will spread from one child to another at school. Examination with a Wood's lamp can be extremely helpful in identifying those affected in an epidemic. *M. canis* is usually limited to the handlers of the affected animal and usually does not spread from human to human. The physical signs are patches of redness and scaling of the scalp with loss of hair (Fig. 3.30). The degree of inflammation with *M. audouinii* may be quite small but can be considerable with *M. canis*, even amounting to kerion formation on occasion.

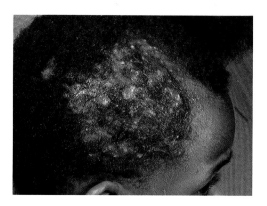

Fig. 3.27 Tinea capitis. There is pronounced weeping and crusting coupled with hair loss in this case of ringworm caught from an infected cat.

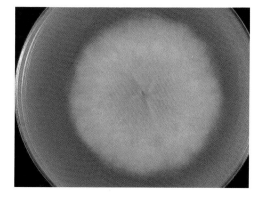

Fig. 3.28 M. canis. On culture, the underside of the plate is yellow. By courtesy of Dr. Y.M. Clayton, St. John's Hospital for Diseases of the Skin.

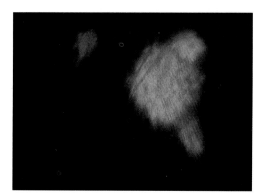

Fig. 3.29 Wood's light fluorescence. *Microsporum* hair infections fluoresce under Wood's light. This is helpful in identifying affected children in epidemics. By courtesy of Dr. Y.M. Clayton, St. John's Hospital for Diseases of the Skin.

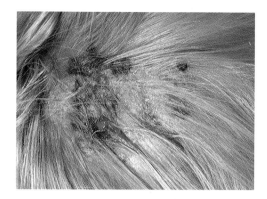

Fig. 3.30 Tinea capitis. In zoophilic infections there is considerable inflammation (kerion) with loss of hair. An infected kitten was the cause in this case.

LARGE-SPORED ECTOTHRIX FUNGI. The zoophilic species of the *Trichophyton* genus are responsible for large-spored ectothrix fungi. *T. verrucosum* is contracted from cattle or horses and *T. mentagrophytes* var. *granulare* from cattle, horses or rodents. The inflammatory response is considerable (Fig. 3.31). There is loss of hair in patches, redness and thick scaling. Kerion formation may occur. These species do not fluoresce with Wood's lamp. The anthropophilic species of the *Trichophyton* genus rarely cause tinea capitis.

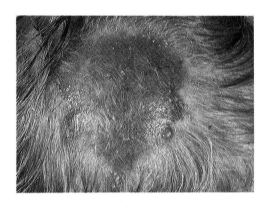

Fig. 3.31 Tinea capitis. Ringworm of the scalp due to animal fungi is characterized by severe inflammation which may result in kerion formation. This adult was infected by a cattle ringworm. Scalp ringworm in adults is very unusual.

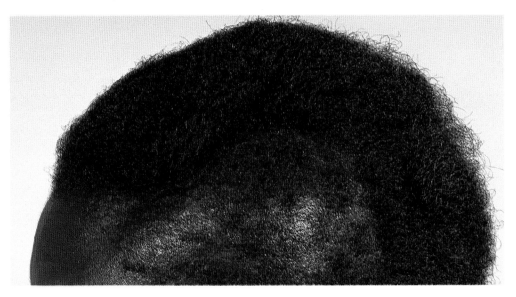

Fig. 3.32 Tinea capitis. *T. soudanense*, an anthropophilic fungus, was responsible for this boy's scalp ringworm. He came from West Africa where he had acquired this endothrix infection.

Endothrix Infections

The hyphae and spores invade the hair shaft and the outer sheath is spared. The hair is completely destroyed down to its base and black dots are left behind. The degree of inflammation is not great and a patchy baldness without much scaling may be all that is to be found on examination. *T. tonsurans (T. sulphureum)*, *T. soudanense* (Fig. 3.32) and *T. violaceum* are the fungi responsible. They are rarely seen in the United Kingdom.

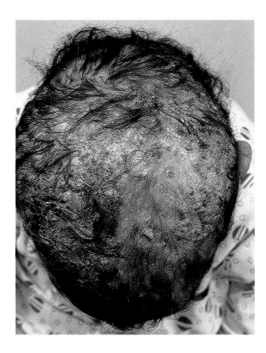

Fig. 3.33 Kerion. There is crusting and the hair is matted secondary to the severe inflammatory reaction. By courtesy of St. John's Hospital for Diseases of the Skin.

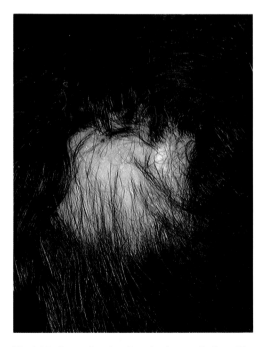

Fig. 3.34 Favus. Scarring alopecia often results from this infection with *T. schoenleinii*.

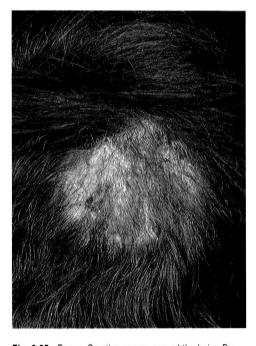

Fig. 3.35 Favus. Crusting occurs around the hairs. By courtesy of St. John's Hospital for Diseases of the Skin.

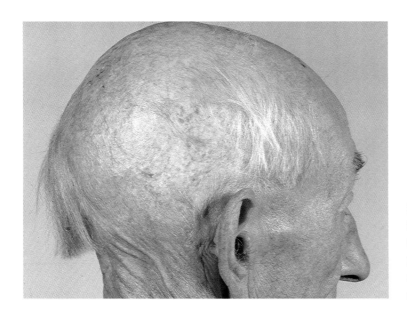

Fig. 3.36 Alopecia secondary to irradiation of scalp ringworm. Scalp ringworm was treated with irradiation before griseofulvin was available. Over-irradiation resulted in life-long alopecia.

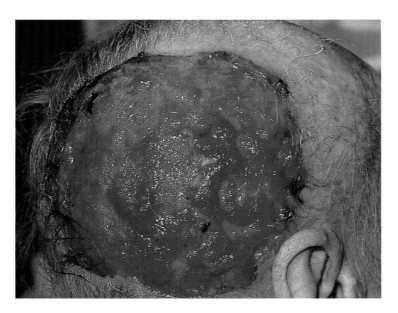

Fig. 3.37 Basal cell carcinoma secondary to irradiation of scalp ringworm. Over-irradiation of scalp ringworm may result in neoplastic change many decades later.

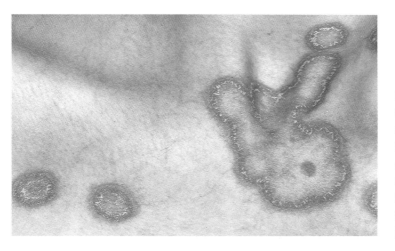

Fig. 3.38 Tinea corporis. The activity of ringworm occurs at the margins of the lesions which have a tendency to heal centrally. Scrapings should be taken from the red scaly margin for the identification of hyphae. By courtesy of Dr. A.C. Pembroke.

Kerion

This is a severe inflammatory scalp reaction to a ringworm infection, usually of animal origin and particularly *T. verrucosum* or *T. mentagrophytes* var. *granulare*. The scalp is a red, warm, painful, pustular mass. There is crusting and the hairs become matted (Fig. 3.33) and fall out. The condition is self-limiting because of the host rejection but permanent scarring and alopecia may ensue if the condition is not treated.

Favus

This is very rare in Western Europe but common in the Middle East. It is important to diagnose this fungal infection immediately because neglect may lead to permanent scarring and thus alopecia (Fig. 3.34). This rarely happens with the other fungi covered here. Favus is caused by *T. schoenleinii*. It is an endothrix infection but the hyphae are not as abundant as in the other endothrix infections so the hair is less damaged and may grow quite long. Classically, small crusts occur around the hairs (Fig. 3.35). These are known as scutulae but they may not always be present. There is a characteristic mousy odour associated with this condition. It is imperative to examine and culture the hairs in any case of patchy alopecia.

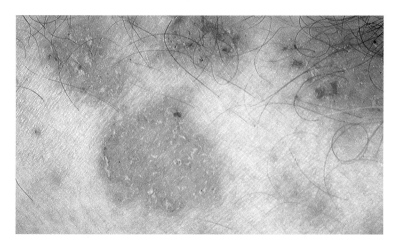

Fig. 3.39 Discoid eczema. The lesions do not show central healing or post-inflammatory pigmentation and are red and scaling across the lesion.

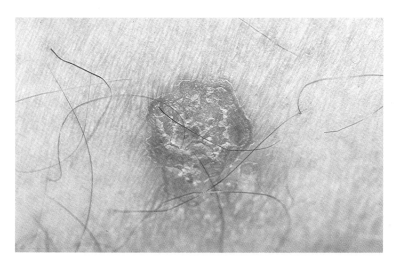

Fig. 3.40 Discoid eczema. The lesions may be crusted in discoid eczema. The activity of the eruption is even across the surface. By courtesy of St. John's Hospital for Diseases of the Skin.

Treatment

Tinea capitis responds well to griseofulvin or ketoconazole. The former has a long, safe track record and is the treatment of choice. Prior to 1958 when griseofulvin became available, treatment of this condition could be far from satisfactory. It was often treated with radiotherapy in order to induce epilation of the affected hairs. Occasionally, particularly in the earlier part of the century when radiation dosages were not very accurate, overdose occurred and permanent alopecia resulted (Fig. 3.36). In some cases, tumours of the head, neck and skin of the scalp have developed fifty or sixty years later (Fig. 3.37).

Tinea Corporis

This is the form of dermatophyte infection which is best described as ringworm (Fig. 3.38). However, the term 'ringworm' is still confusing because many common skin disorders, for example discoid eczema (Figs. 3.39 and 3.40) and the herald patch of pityriasis rosea (Fig. 3.41) are ring-shaped whereas dermatophyte infections may not be ring-shaped.

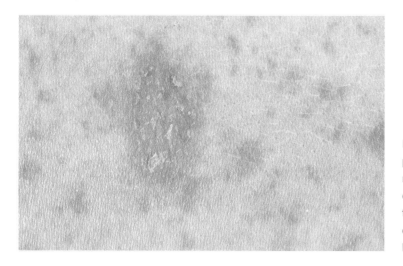

Fig. 3.41 The herald patch of pityriasis rosea. This is often misdiagnosed as tinea but the erythema remains constant throughout the lesion. A few days later other small oval pink lesions develop.

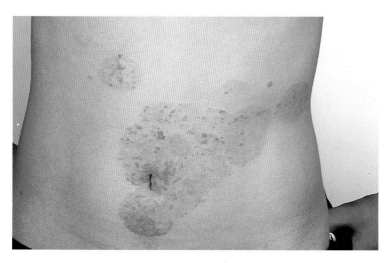

Fig. 3.42 Tinea corporis. Post-inflammatory hyperpigmentation is a feature of healing tinea. This eruption had been misdiagnosed and treated with topical steroids which reduce the inflammatory response.

The features which suggest tinea corporis are an annular eruption, with a tendency to active margins and a healing central area which is often hyperpigmented (Fig. 3.42). The fungus tends to migrate outwards for fresh nutrient material. The lesions are red and scaly and asymmetrically placed (Fig. 3.43). The degree of erythema and scaling depends on the type of fungus. Animal ringworm is much more inflammatory than human ringworm (Fig. 3.44).

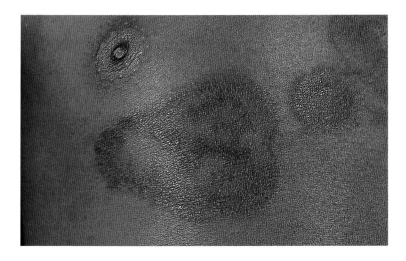

Fig. 3.43 Tinea corporis. The margin of the annular lesions is most active. The lesions are asymmetrically distributed.

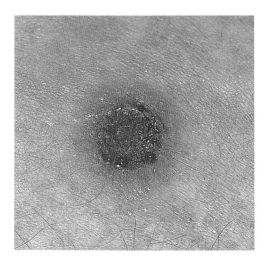

Fig. 3.44 Tinea corporis. Animal ringworm infections are more inflammatory than human. *Microsporum canis* was grown on culturing scales from this lesion.

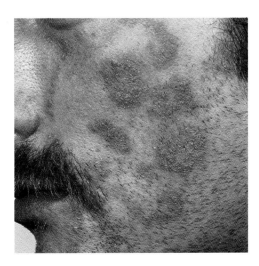

Fig. 3.45 Tinea of the face. Annular, red, scaly patches are present on the cheek. The condition had been misdiagnosed and treated with topical steroids which caused the eruption to spread.

Tinea Faciei

Tinea of the face has much the same characteristics as tinea corporis. The lesions are asymmetrical, annular red patches. There is scaling and redness at the periphery of each lesion (Fig. 3.45) and a tendency towards central healing and pigmentation (Fig. 3.46).

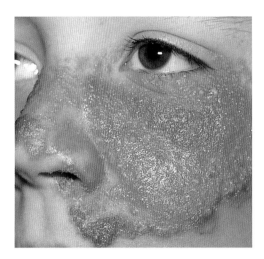

Fig. 3.46 Tinea of the face. The margin of the eruption is most active. Many pustules are present (kerion) as a result of mistreatment with topical steroids.

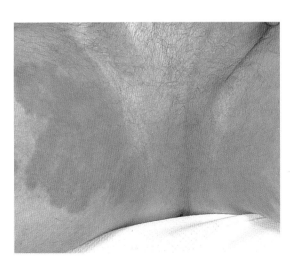

Fig. 3.47 Tinea cruris. The margins of the eruption on the thighs are red and there is post-inflammatory pigmentation in areas which have been invaded by the fungus.

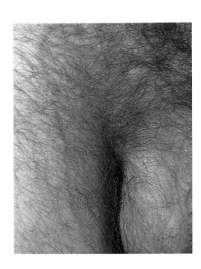

Fig. 3.48 Tinea cruris. The margin of the eruption is red and scaling and tends to advance away from the genito-crural fold down the inner thigh. By courtesy of St. John's Hospital for Diseases of the Skin.

Tinea Cruris

Ringworm in the groin is a common pruritic eruption in young men but is unusual in women. It is caused by the anthropophilic fungi only, particularly *Trichophyton rubrum*, *Epidermophyton floccosum* and *T. mentagrophytes* var. *interdigitale*. It spreads outwards asymmetrically from the genito-crural folds and down the thigh, leaving post-inflammatory pigmentation (Fig. 3.47). The advancing border is well-defined, slightly raised, red and scaly (Fig. 3.48). It is frequently misdiagnosed and treated with topical glucocorticosteroids which permit the condition to spread (Figs. 3.49 and 3.50). It is, therefore,

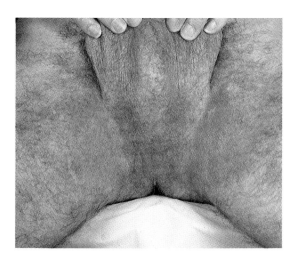

Fig. 3.49 Tinea cruris (tinea incognito). The eruption is frequently misdiagnosed and treated with topical steroids which suppress the physical signs of inflammation so that the linear border is not visible. Scrapings were, however, full of hyphae.

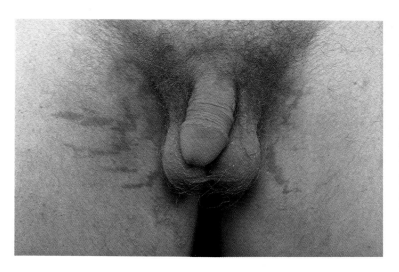

Fig. 3.50 Tinea cruris (tinea incognito). This had been treated with powerful topical steroids. Gross striae have resulted but the inflammatory physical signs are suppressed except for an active red and scaling edge in the lower part of the right inner thigh, where the patient has failed to apply the steroid. By courtesy of St. John's Hospital for Diseases of the Skin.

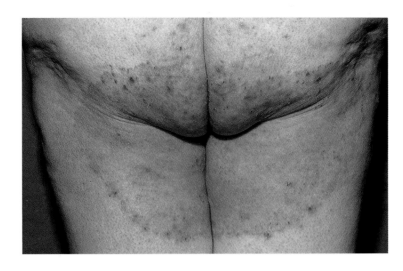

Fig. 3.51 Tinea of the buttocks. Tinea may spread from the groin onto the buttocks, especially if treated with topical steroids. The active edge is pronounced with central hyperpigmentation. There is considerable excoriation because tinea may be very pruritic in this area.

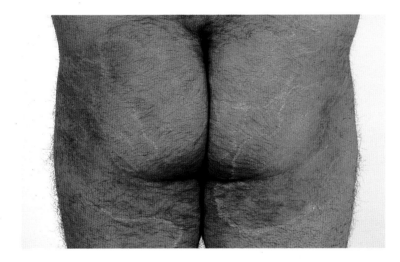

Fig. 3.52 Tinea of the buttocks. This man also had sarcoidosis and the accompanying immunosuppression permitted the rash to become extensive. *E. floccosum* was grown on cultures of his skin.

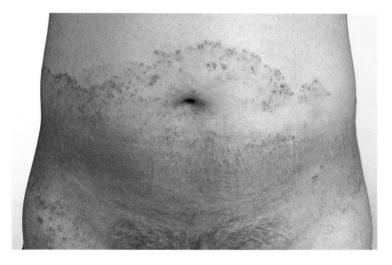

Fig. 3.53 Tinea of the lower abdomen. This man had a *T. rubrum* infection of the groin which had been treated with topical steroids and had become extensive.

always wise to examine scrapings from any skin condition in the groin for the presence of fungi. There may well be evidence of tinea elsewhere, especially in the toe webs and toenails which may lead to recurrent attacks unless treated. The eruption may spread onto the buttocks (Figs. 3.51 and 3.52) and lower abdomen (Fig. 3.53).

Tinea Pedis

This is colloquially known as 'athlete's foot'. It is more common in men and is usually acquired from communal changing rooms in institutions or sports facilities. Only the anthropophilic fungi are responsible. *T. mentagrophytes* var. *interdigitale* and *E. floccosum* produce similar clinical appearances but *T. rubrum* is described separately because of its special characteristics.

The eruption is found in the toe webs. There is peeling, scaling and erythema. The skin is macerated (Fig. 3.54). The condition is itchy but may become sore if it is fissured (Fig. 3.55). The eruption is usually

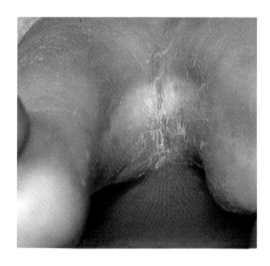

Fig. 3.54 Tinea pedis. The eruption starts as maceration between the toes.

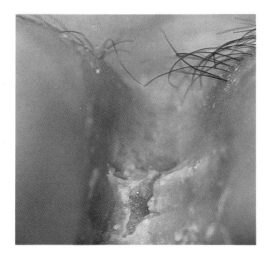

Fig. 3.55 Tinea pedis. Painful fissuring may occur in addition to the maceration. By courtesy of St. John's Hospital for Diseases of the Skin.

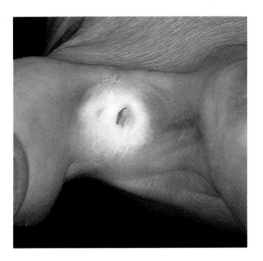

Fig. 3.56 Soft corn. Corns due to friction between the skin of the fourth and fifth toes due to ill-fitting shoes are sometimes misdiagnosed as tinea pedis.

asymmetrical, one foot being more involved than the other. Many individuals have this condition between the webs of their fourth and fifth toes but only about a quarter of these cases are due to tinea. Most cases are due to compression of the fourth toe against the fifth by tight-fitting shoes, thus producing a macerated intertrigo, but no fungi will be recovered on culture of the skin scales. This condition may respond to toe spacers and better fitting footwear. Equally, soft corns (Figs. 3.56 and 3.57) caused by the rubbing of the fourth toe against the fifth secondary to ill-fitting shoes are regularly mistaken for tinea. However, infection of other toe webs is almost certainly due to tinea.

The condition spreads onto the sole of the foot and presents as an itchy, vesicular eruption (Figs. 3.58 and 3.59), usually unilaterally. The vesicles often coalesce and large confluent blisters result. In these acute, vesiculo-bullous eruptions, secondary bacterial infection may be superimposed and a lymphangiitis results. Occasionally, a vesicular eruption identical to that of an acute hand eczema (pompholyx) may result along the sides of the fingers (Fig. 3.60) and hands. This is referred to as an 'id' phenomenon. No fungi are recovered from these vesicles but the eruption does respond to treatment of the tinea pedis.

If tinea is untreated or mistreated with topical steroids it may spread onto the dorsa of the feet. The eruption is asymmetrical (Figs. 3.61 and 3.62) and tends to have an active red scaling margin (Fig. 3.63).

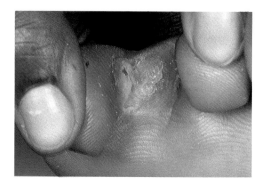

Fig. 3.57 Soft corn. The skin is thickened and hyperkeratotic. Only the lateral side of the web is involved.

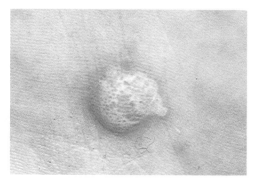

Fig. 3.58 Tinea pedis. Tinea may present as vesicles on the sole of the foot. The eruption is usually unilateral.

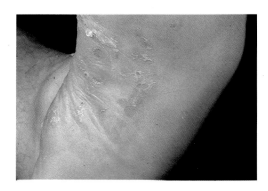

Fig. 3.59 Tinea pedis. Vesicles and scaling are present on the sole of the foot. This is often colloquially known as 'athlete's foot'.

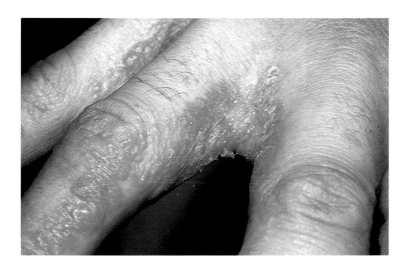

Fig. 3.60 Pompholyx. Acute eczema of the hand may occasionally result as a reaction to an acute tinea pedis (an 'id' phenomenon).

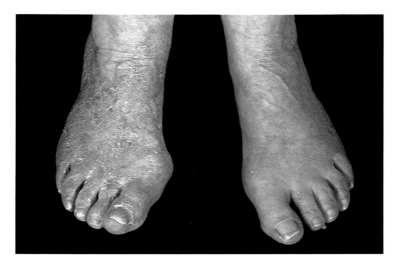

Fig. 3.61 Tinea pedis. The eruption is often unilateral. The toenails are also involved. Topical steroids were responsible for the spread of the rash.

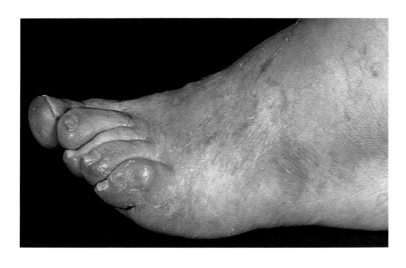

Fig. 3.62 Tinea pedis. The tendency to red rings is visible. The toenails are involved.

This is now the commonest dermatophyte infection in the United Kingdom (Fig. 3.64). It was rare before World War II but was imported by British troops who acquired it in the Far East. It commences, as do the other fungi, between the toes, causing macerated, fissured and scaling skin, but does not cause a vesicular response on the soles. The host's response is minimal so the degree of inflammatory change is correspondingly small.

Thus, the changes on the skin may be quite subtle (Fig. 3.65). The skin is dry and rather powdery, particularly in the skin creases and there is a peeling of the skin. Nail involvement is frequent and the fungus may subsequently spread to the hands and fingernails. Tinea cruris is very common. *T. rubrum* lesions may spread to the lower legs and produce a papular or nodular eruption on the calf or shin. The condition is known as Majocchi's granuloma (Fig. 3.66).

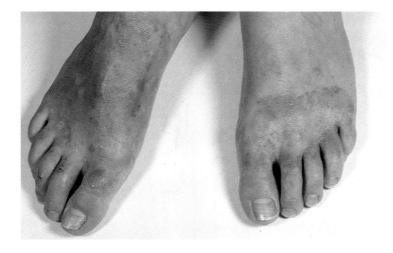

Fig. 3.63 Tinea pedis. This man had been prescribed a powerful topical glucocorticosteroid. The condition had spread considerably. The asymmetry of the eruption is suggestive of tinea.

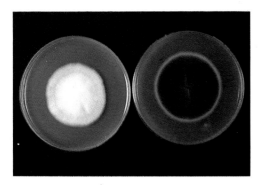

Fig. 3.64 *Trichophyton rubrum.* The underside of the plate is a red colour, hence the adjective rubrum. It is the most common cause of dermatophyte infections in the United Kingdom. By courtesy of Dr. Y.M. Clayton, St. John's Hospital for Diseases of the Skin.

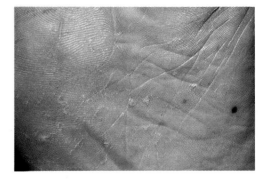

Fig. 3.65 T. rubrum infection of the feet. The condition presents as peeling of the skin.

Tinea Manuum

Ringworm of the dorsum of the hand or wrist (Figs. 3.67 and 3.68) should be regarded as a form of tinea corporis, but ringworm of the palm presents special characteristics. It is almost invariably caused by *T. rubrum*. It is unilateral and may remain this way for decades, a situation for which there is no satisfactory explanation at the present time. There are crescentic, peeling scales (Fig. 3.69) to be seen and a powdery filling-in of the skin creases (Fig. 3.70). The palmar skin feels dry. Sooner or later the fingernails become involved.

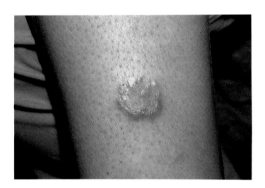

Fig. 3.66 Majocchi's granuloma. This is a nodular annular eruption on the back of the calf due to *T. rubrum*.

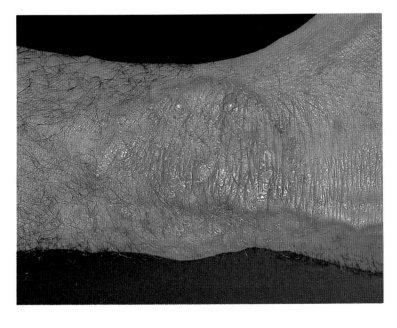

Fig. 3.67 Tinea of the wrist. The eruption is annular with central healing.

Tinea Incognito

This is an artificial term to describe ringworm infections that have been misdiagnosed and treated with topical glucocorticosteroids. The use of topical steroids somewhat modifies the clinical picture of the eruption because there is a damping down of the usual inflammatory responses which indicate the presence of the disorder. Thus the margin of the eruption, which is usually slightly raised, red and scaly, may be barely perceptible. There may, however, be an untreated area which will suggest the correct diagnosis. It is imperative to take scrapings from any eruption with scales, particularly those which do not conform to the correct pattern of a skin disorder.

Tinea Unguium

The nails are often invaded by the anthropophilic fungi, especially *T. rubrum*.

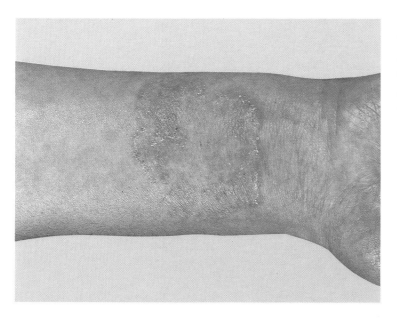

Fig. 3.68 Tinea of the wrist. This is frequently misdiagnosed as contact dermatitis to a wrist-watch but the red scaly margin and central healing suggest tinea.

MANAGEMENT OF DERMATOPHYTE INFECTIONS

Griseofulvin was a major advance in the management of dermatophyte infections. It is a very safe drug and patients only occasionally experience side-effects, nausea and headaches being the most common. It is the only effective treatment for ringworm of the scalp and nails and for *T. rubrum* infections. Tinea corporis, tinea pedis and tinea cruris will show some response to topical anti-fungal agents such as the imidazoles and half-strength Whitfield's ointment but they are not as efficient as griseofulvin. Most cases will clear within four weeks of treatment with griseofulvin but nail involvement represents a special case. Ketoconazole is also effective but in view of its hepatotoxicity, it is a second line drug.

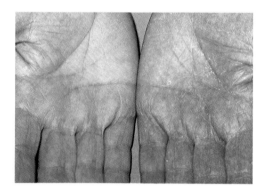

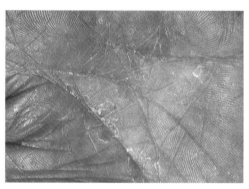

Fig. 3.69   T. rubrum infection of the hand. The eruption is invariably unilateral. Closer examination reveals crescentic peeling scales.

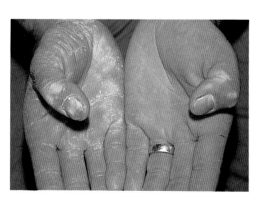

Fig. 3.70   Tinea of the hands. The eruption is unilateral and often remains so indefinitely. Note the involvement of the thumbnail.

4
Infestations of the Skin

SCABIES

Scabies is a common, intensely itchy disorder of the skin caused by an acarus or mite, *Sarcoptes scabei* var. *hominis* (Fig. 4.1). It is simple to diagnose and eminently treatable.

The mite is capable of crawling from one human skin to another but it does require relatively prolonged contact between the two. The condition is caught from a bedfellow where intimate contact is likely, but not from momentary contact between adults, such as shaking hands. However, the infection is readily transmitted between children where protracted physical contact is commonplace. Children, particularly infants, are constantly handled by adults and infection may easily be transmitted.

The pregnant female mite, having established herself on the skin of a new victim, will burrow into the horny layer of the skin and lay her eggs. The preferred sites for this are areas where the stratum corneum (horny layer) is at its thickest – for example, the palms and soles. Once infection has taken place it may be a month or two before the symptoms of pruritus commence. Although the burrows will be visible, they will not be noticed by the patients in the absence of symptoms; indeed, it is rare for a patient to note their rather distinctive morphology. This incubation period is important, as it enables a time to be calculated when the patient may have contracted the infection, so that contacts may be identified and treated.

The cardinal symptom is of itching all over the body, which is particularly intense at night or after a warm bath. It begins slowly at first but gradually becomes intense and often unbearable, driving the patient to distraction and inability to sleep at nights.

The diagnostic physical sign is the burrow (Figs. 4.2 and 4.3). This is a serpiginous track which is just palpable and about 10mm long. The mite is only just visible to the human eye as a minute white dot at the end of the track. It can be extracted with a needle and demonstrated under the microscope. The most common sites for the burrows are the hands, particularly along the sides of the fingers, in the web between the thumb and the first finger (Fig. 4.4), and at the wrist overlying the hypo- and hyperthenar

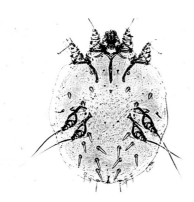

Fig. 4.1 Scabies. Scabies is caused by an acarus or mite, *Sarcoptes scabei* var. *hominis*. It burrows into the skin but may be extracted with a needle and identified under a light microscope.

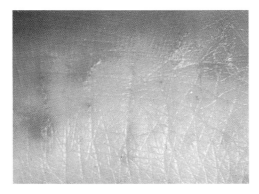

Fig. 4.2 Scabies. Linear, slightly raised serpiginous lesions (burrows) are diagnostic of scabies. By courtesy of St. Mary's Hospital.

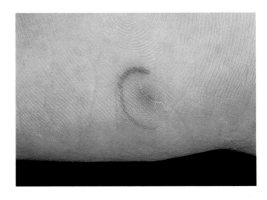

Fig. 4.3 Scabies. Linear burrows occur most often on the palmar surfaces.

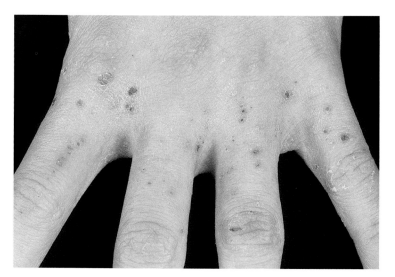

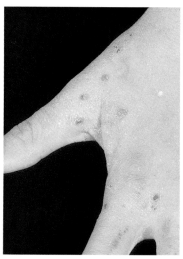

Fig. 4.4 Scabies. Papules and burrows occur between the fingers, especially in the web between the thumb and the index finger.

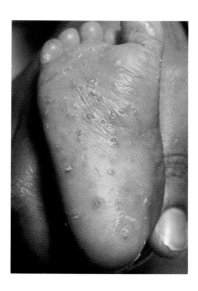

Fig. 4.5 Scabies. Papules and burrows occur on the soles and sides of the feet. Children are particularly affected in this manner.

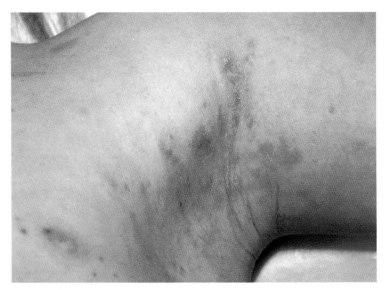

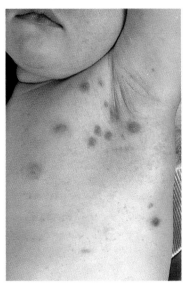

Fig. 4.6 Scabies. Papules commonly occur in the axillae (above) and nodules may develop (left).

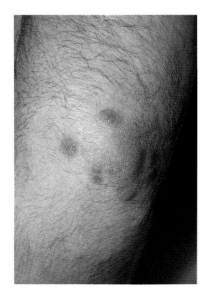

Fig. 4.7 Scabies. Nodules around the elbows are characteristic.

eminences. The plantar surfaces are particularly involved in children (Fig. 4.5). These lesions are diagnostic because they appear in no other disease. The burrow may develop into an inflammatory papule or nodule in the anterior axillary folds (Fig. 4.6), the points of the elbows (Fig. 4.7) and the genitalia. Indeed, papules on the penis or the scrotum in an itching patient are highly suspicious of scabies (Figs. 4.8–4.10).

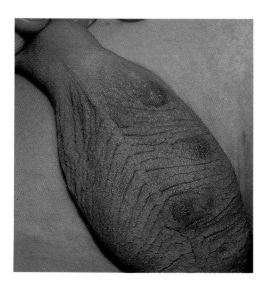

Fig. 4.8 Scabies. Genital papules are almost diagnostic of scabies.

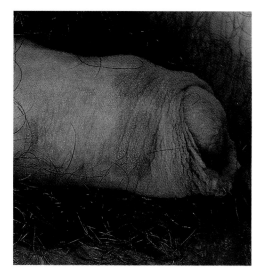

Fig. 4.9 Scabies. Nodules may persist on the genitalia for many weeks after the disease has been treated.

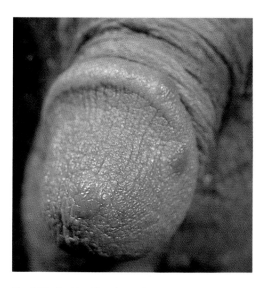

Fig. 4.10 Scabies. Papules on the scrotum or penis are an almost universal finding in males with scabies. By courtesy of St. Mary's Hospital.

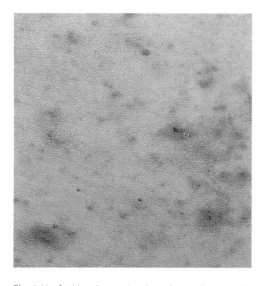

Fig. 4.11 Scabies. An excoriated papular eruption occurs in addition to the burrows.

Once sensitization to the presence of the mite has occurred, a papular and urticarial eruption (Fig. 4.11) occurs on the trunk (Figs. 4.12–4.13), buttocks, inner thighs and forearms. Lesions are not seen on the face. Excoriations and bruising are commonplace as a result of scratching.

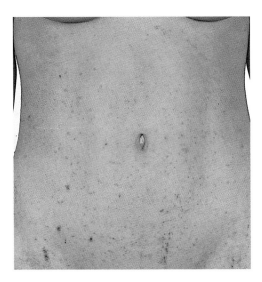

Fig. 4.12 Scabies. This is an intensely pruritic condition. After an incubation period of approximately one month, generalized itching occurs, with a fine papular eruption on the trunk.

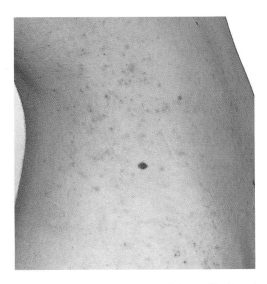

Fig. 4.13 Scabies. Widespread excoriations and bruising of the skin occur.

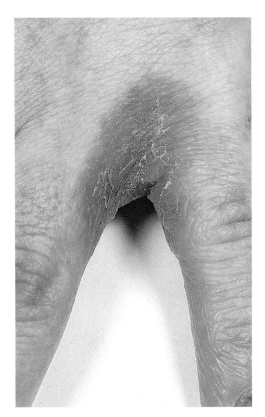

Fig. 4.14 Eczema. Eczema between the fingers is sometimes misdiagnosed as scabies or vice-versa.

The extent of physical signs depends to a large extent on the personal hygiene of the patient, so that in the well-washed only one or two burrows may be found, although the pruritus will be just as intense. The scabies mite has no respect of status, so the condition is found in all social classes, contrary to popular belief. Sometimes the condition becomes secondarily infected, particularly in childhood, but this is not the rule – a surprising fact in view of the intensity of the scratching of the skin.

Very occasionally, extremely extensive infestation with acari occurs, so-called Norwegian or crusted scabies. This condition occurs in immunosuppressed patients. Institutionalized individuals with Down's syndrome are also prone to this, perhaps because they have disordered immunological function or possibly because they may not scratch and therefore eliminate a certain proportion of the mites mechanically. In recent years, patients have been misdiagnosed as having eczema (Fig. 4.14) and treated with powerful topical steroids (Fig. 4.15). These are immunosuppressive and allow easy dissemination of the mites. The diagnosis of Norwegian scabies is usually made after members of staff of an institution develop scabies in an epidemic form, as this variety of scabies is highly infectious requiring the minimum of contact. A myriad of burrows will be found on close examination of the skin, particularly on the hands, but the most striking feature is the degree of crusting and scaling of the skin. This may be virtually universal, including the face, but will predominate in those areas where the eruption of ordinary scabies is usually found, for example between the fingers (Fig. 4.16).

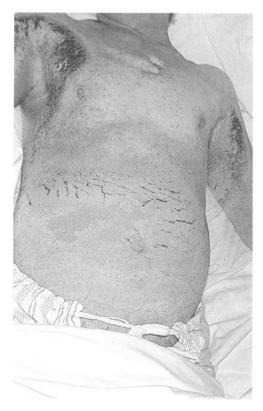

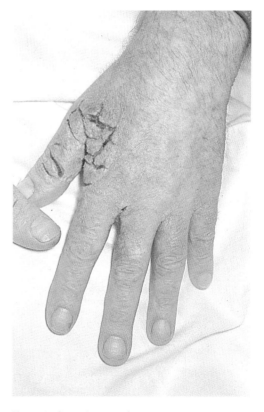

Fig. 4.15 Crusted (Norwegian) scabies. This man was misdiagnosed as having eczema and was admitted to hospital where he was treated with powerful topical and eventually systemic steroids. The correct diagnosis was made when several other patients, nurses and doctors developed irritation of the skin. This man was located as the source. By courtesy of St. Mary's Hospital.

Fig. 4.16 Crusted scabies. Crusting is present between the finger webs. The lesions were teeming with acari and were therefore highly infectious. The condition responded rapidly to routine treatment with Quellada. By courtesy of St. Mary's Hospital.

Scabies is easily treated, but the treatment must be done thoroughly and conscientiously, and some time must be spent in explaining this to the patient; otherwise treatment failures will occur. Gamma benzene hexachloride should be applied from the neck downwards to all parts of the body and this should be emphasized so that the soles of the feet, the hands, between the fingers, the genitalia and the natal cleft are all included. The treatment should be applied by the patient or a parent after a hot bath and allowed to dry for five minutes. Twenty-four hours later a second application is made after another bath. All members of the family and contacts should be treated, whether or not they have begun to itch.

It should be explained to the patient that the itching will not go away immediately, although it will usually diminish in intensity. This is important because the patient may be tempted to use the acaricidal lotion repeatedly. These lotions, especially benzyl benzoate, are primary irritants of the skin and will frequently lead to an eczematous eruption. The patient will itch as a consequence of this eczema; re-application of the lotions will only make the situation worse. Benzyl benzoate should probably no longer be used to treat scabies. It is important to follow the patient's progress because it may be necessary to prescribe a topical steroid to overcome the eczema resulting from the treatment. It is not uncommon for a patient to have pruritus for up to four weeks after successful treatment. Once a patient has had an attack of scabies it is most unlikely that it will occur again. On subsequent contact with the scabies mite the body mounts an immediate immune response to the acarus which is then unable to get a foothold. It is a myth that scabies can be contracted from infected clothing since the mite lives in the skin and not on the clothing. There is therefore no need to take any special measures regarding clothing or bedding.

PEDICULOSIS

There are three varieties of louse which can be distinguished morphologically and which have a predilection for certain sites on the body. The head louse is elongated in shape, as is the body louse, but the latter is larger. The crab louse is shorter and is as broad as it is long; its name derives from the crab-like claws on the rear legs with which it grasps hair. Lice have six legs, are wingless and give rise to symptoms of irritation of the skin. Unlike the acarus, no immunity is developed to the louse and repeated infections may occur.

Pediculosis Capitis

Infestation of the scalp, particularly in children of school age, is still remarkably common. The lice are obvious to the naked eye on examination and may be seen to move. The eggs, which are known as nits, are seen attached to the hairs (Fig. 4.17). These can be distinguished from dandruff by the fact that nits cannot be shaken off the hair although they can be slid up the shaft and then pulled off. Secondary infection and lymphadenopathy often occur as a result of scratching. Because resistance to gamma benzene hexachloride has been reported, 0.5% malathion lotion is applied to the scalp and left on for 24 hours. The nits should be removed with a fine tooth comb and the treatment repeated after ten days. It is important that other members of the family and the rest of the children at the school are examined, otherwise infection can obviously recur. The condition is far more common in children because they are more likely to be in fairly close physical contact, although adults can also be affected.

Pediculosis Pubis

The crab louse (*Phthirus pubis*) is found primarily in the pubic area but also, especially in a hirsute individual, on the limbs, chest, in the axillae and even on the eyebrows or eyelashes but not on the scalp. The infection is usually transmitted sexually. The condition gives rise to intense pruritus. The crab louse can easily be identified with the naked eye and can often be seen to be moving. The nits are attached to the hairs and can be confirmed under a microscope. Treatment is with gamma benzene hexachloride applied thoroughly to all the affected areas. The application should be repeated ten days later to deal with any eggs which may have hatched out since the first application. Although *Phthirus pubis* lives primarily on the skin, it may be found on the underclothing and it is wise to examine this for evidence of lice and disinfect with DDT if necessary.

Pediculosis Corporis

Body lice are rarely seen in normal individuals, except under disaster conditions when there is chaos, overcrowding and a breakdown in hygiene. Vagrants, however, are frequently infested. These pediculi differ from the others in that although they feed off the skin, they breed and live in the clothing, including the bed clothing of the infested individual. They are found in the seams of the underclothing

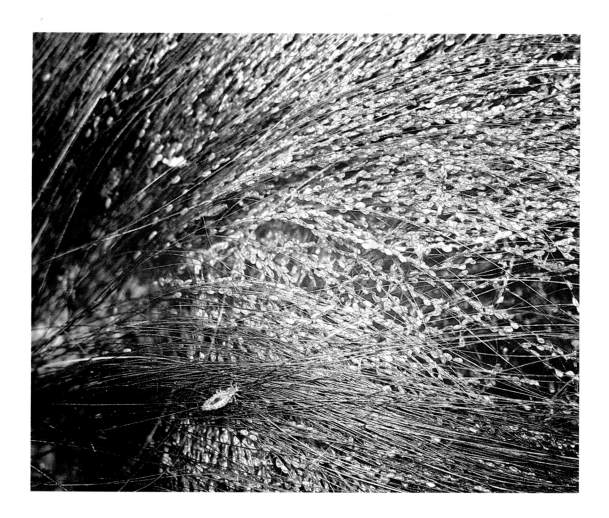

Fig. 4.17 Pediculosis capitis. A mass of nits and pediculi are present in this man's hair. A louse is clearly visible.
By courtesy of St. Bartholomew's Hospital.

and cause extremely intense pruritus in the skin closest to the clothes such as the shoulders, neck, breasts, and around the buttocks. Secondary sepsis is common. Since repeated infection is commonplace in the lodging houses which vagrants frequent, chronic infestation ensues because there is no natural immunity. As a result of continual scratching, the skin becomes pigmented, thickened, dry and scaly; a situation known colloquially as 'vagabond's disease'. Under certain conditions the body louse may carry Rickettsia and result in typhus, trench or relapsing fevers.

The diagnosis of body lice is remarkably easy, provided the condition is considered and a search is made of the clothing. Treatment with gamma benzene hexachloride alone will not cure the patient: he must be separated from the infested clothing and have a fresh set provided. The infested clothing should be fumigated, DDT is effective.

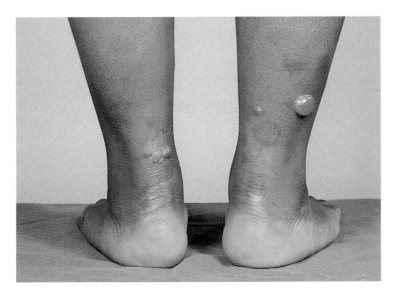

Fig. 4.18 Insect bites. Urticarial papular, bullous and post-inflammatory pigmented lesions are present in this West Indian child.

Fig. 4.19 Insect bites. A central punctum is sometimes visible within an urticarial lesion. By courtesy of St. John's Hospital for Diseases of the Skin.

INSECT BITES

These are extremely common and must be considered in the differential diagnosis of any patient complaining of itching. Urticarial wheals (Fig. 4.18), often with a central punctum (Fig. 4.19), papules, vesicles and less commonly blisters (Fig. 4.20) amid excoriations may suggest the diagnosis. The lesions are usually scattered asymmetrically over the body, or concentrated on the lower legs (Fig. 4.21). The source requires detection and careful consideration of the personal habits of the patient. Thus, pets may house fleas or mites, as may homes previously occupied by pets. Recently acquired old furniture may be

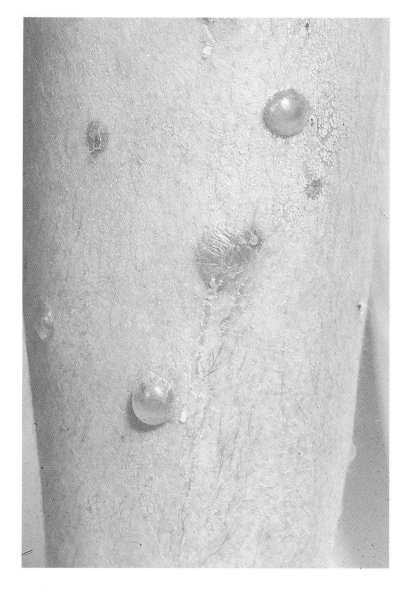

Fig. 4.20 Insect bites. Bullae sometimes develop, especially on the lower legs. By courtesy of St. Mary's Hospital.

the residence of bugs. Trips abroad or to the country, or work in the garden may bring the patient into contact with a host of insects including mosquitoes, caterpillars (Fig. 4.22), ticks and sandflies. These, in addition to causing bites, may harbour disease; for example, malaria (mosquitoes), Rocky Mountain spotted fever (ticks), and leishmaniasis (sandflies). The fact that only certain individuals seem to be attractive to insects and other members of the household or party may be spared, may incline the patient to discount insects when considering the diagnosis.

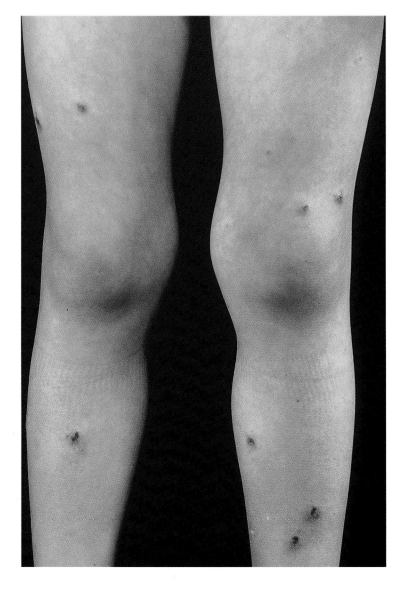

Fig. 4.21 Insect bites. The lower legs are a very common site. Bites are intensely pruritic and therefore excoriated. By courtesy of St. John's Hospital for Diseases of the Skin.

Domestic animals, especially cats and dogs, are responsible for many cases of unsuspected insect bites. The owners find it hard to believe that their pet could acquire an infestation. Fleas constitute the majority of ectoparasites living on pets. They breed in cracks and crevices in floorboards, amongst soft furnishings, in dust and dirt and they particularly enjoy centrally-heated, and fitted-carpet environments. The lesions seen on humans are usually grouped, often three at a time in a linear arrangement (Fig. 4.23) on the trunk or limbs. The eruption may become extremely widespread. It causes intense irritation.

Cheyletiella are mites which particularly favour cats and dogs as carriers, but cause them no symptoms. They attack man causing urticarial or papulo-vesicular eruptions. The distribution usually occurs when the animal is held in contact with the human, that is, in the lap area or the lower chest and abdomen, the forearms and thighs.

Animals may acquire scabies (sarcoptic mange). There is no incubation period and burrows are not usually found as in human scabies. The eruption occurs on the parts of the body which have been in

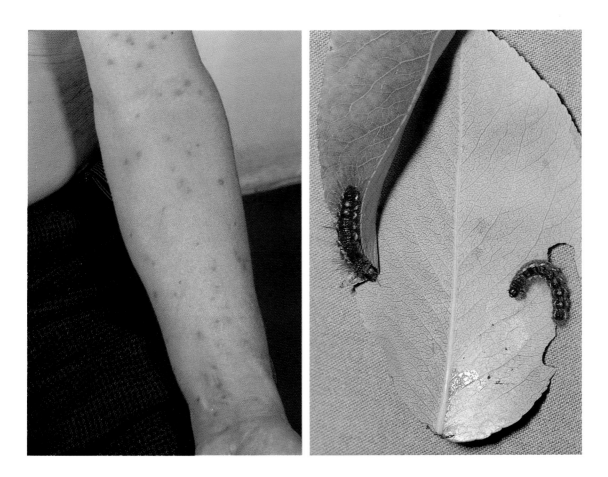

Fig. 4.22 Insect bites. These bites were found to be caused by caterpillars of the brown tail moth.

contact with the infested animal, usually the arms. It has a red papular morphology and is very itchy.

Bedbugs live in crevices in furniture and walls, and usually produce more inflammation than fleas. They must be suspected if the patient has acquired furniture, particularly a bed, or has moved into new lodgings prior to the appearance of the bite. The bugs shun the light and come out at night feeding particularly on exposed areas, such as the arms and face, i.e. parts not covered by night attire or bedclothing. The lesions may be quite substantial (Fig. 4.24) and blood may be found on the clothing the following morning. Many patients will sleep through an attack. The patient may feel quite unwell with a fever, secondary infection (Fig. 4.25) and sometimes lymphadenopathy, especially with recurrent attacks. It is wise to contact public health officials to eradicate the problem.

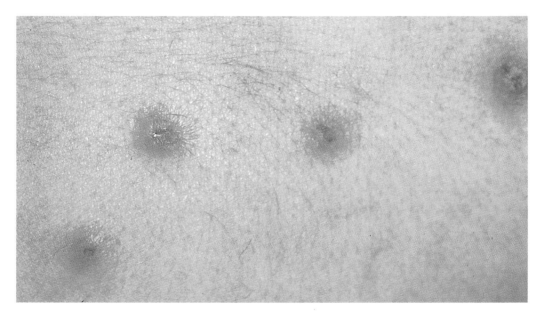

Fig. 4.23 Insect bites. Excoriated papules occurring in linear groups of three or four are characteristic. By courtesy of St. John's Hospital for Diseases of the Skin.

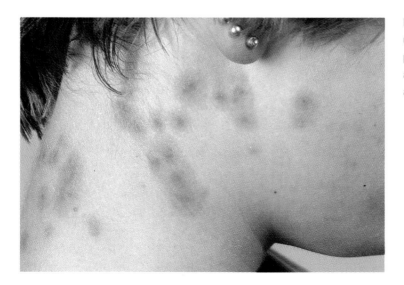

Fig. 4.24 Insect bites. Large urticarial wheals with a central punctum are present on the neck and face. Bed bugs frequently attack exposed areas at night.

Management of Insect Bites

It is helpful to collect brushings from suspect animals onto the shiny surface of brown paper and have these examined by a parasitologist. The finding of evidence of ectoparasites helps to convince the patient of the diagnosis. The animal should be treated by a veterinary surgeon. It is often necessary to fumigate the rooms used by the animal. Occasionally it is necessary to contact public health departments for further investigation.

The patient may be helped by calamine or topical steroids. Secondary infection should be treated with antibiotics.

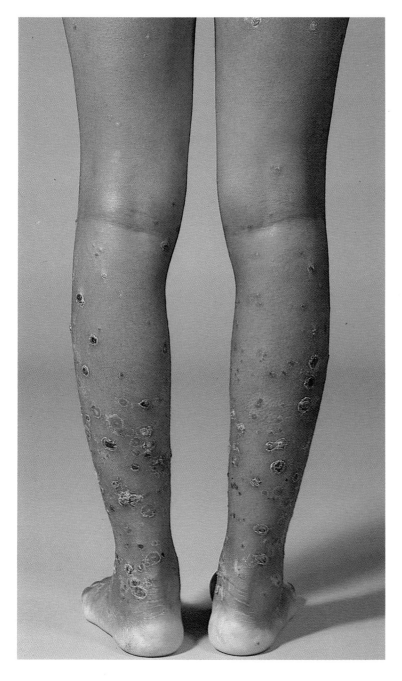

Fig. 4.25 Insect bites.
Secondary infection is common.

5

Tropical Infections of the Skin

LEPROSY (HANSEN'S DISEASE)

This is a chronic infection due to *Mycobacterium leprae* which produces physical signs principally in the skin and nervous tissue. The degree of involvement in either site depends largely on the immunological status of the patient and the bacteriological load. The socio-economic conditions and racial background of the patient are important contributory factors. The disease is transmitted by inhalation or ingestion of infected nasal droplets. The organism invades the Schwann cells which surround the cutaneous nerves. The various types of leprosy are arbitrarily divided into tuberculoid, borderline and lepromatous, based on the immunological status of the patient. These types are known as TT, BB and LL and the intermediate types between these are designated BT and BL. This immunological classification is determined on the basis of the clinical signs and the lepromin test (Fig. 5.1). This is the reaction to an intradermal injection of a standard extract of leprosy tissue. It is positive in tuberculoid leprosy and negative in lepromatous leprosy.

Leprosy is a disorder of tropical countries, particularly India, Africa, South-east Asia and South America. It is uncommon in Western societies. Clearly, it presents most frequently in the skin and only the cutaneous physical signs are described here. However, it is a complex disorder in immunological terms and its management requires considerable skill if nervous tissue function is to be preserved. It is thus usually treated by leprologists.

Tuberculoid Leprosy

The immunological resistance to the leprosy bacillus is high at this end of the spectrum. The skin lesions are few and asymmetrically distributed. The patches are well-defined and often annular in shape (Fig. 5.2). They are red with central hypopigmentation (Fig. 5.3). The surface is dry and scaly, does not

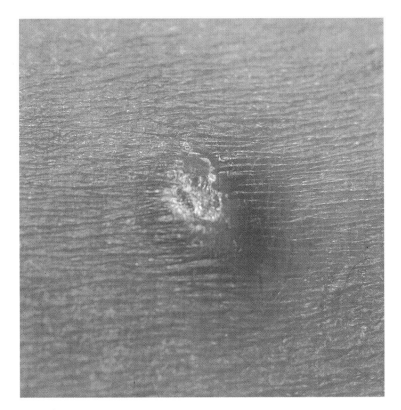

Fig. 5.1 Mitsuda (lepromin) test. This is a reaction to an intradermal injection of a standard extract of leprosy tissue. It is positive in tuberculoid leprosy but negative in lepromatous leprosy. By courtesy of St. John's Hospital for Diseases of the Skin.

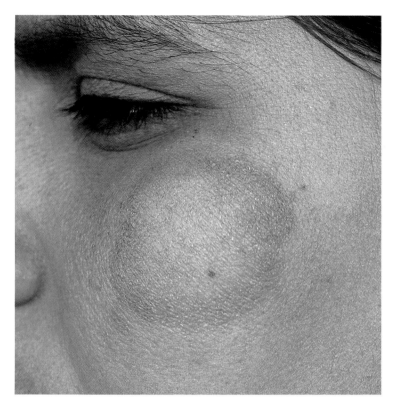

Fig. 5.2 Tuberculoid leprosy. There is a dry, annular, anaesthetic patch on the cheek. Skin biopsy established the diagnosis. By courtesy of St. John's Hospital for Diseases of the Skin.

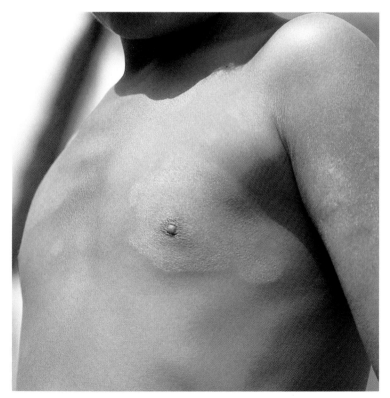

Fig. 5.3 Tuberculoid leprosy. Annular, anaesthetic, hypopigmented patches occur.

sweat and is anaesthetic. The sites of predilection are the cool, peripheral parts of the body such as the face, buttocks, the elbows and knees (Fig. 5.4) and extensor surfaces of the limbs (Fig. 5.5). The peripheral nerves particularly the great auricular, ulnar and peroneal become involved in addition to nervous tissue within the skin lesion. These nerves are thickened and therefore palpable. Involvement leads to a peripheral neuropathy with sensory changes resulting in ulceration of the digits and motor changes in palsies such as footdrop or ulnar nerve paralysis. Skin biopsy will confirm the diagnosis (Fig. 5.6). Non-caseating granulomata are found but bacilli are conspicuously few or likely to be absent.

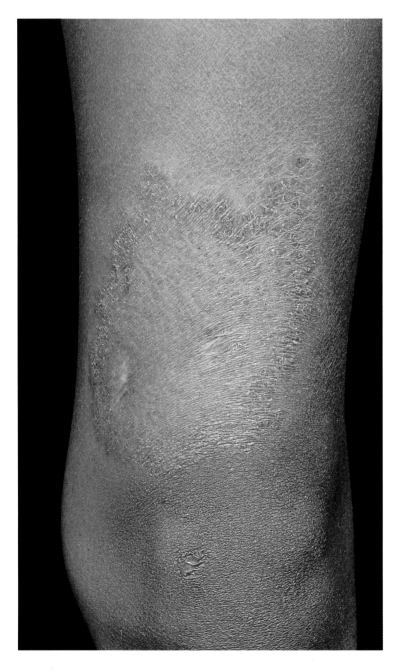

Fig. 5.4 Tuberculoid leprosy. Annular, dry, slightly scaly patches are characteristic. The extensor surface of the knee is a common site. By courtesy of St. John's Hospital for Diseases of the Skin.

Borderline Leprosy

This disorder is a mixture of both tuberculoid and lepromatous leprosy. It is, however, immunologically unstable and can downgrade to lepromatous leprosy or can reverse to tuberculoid leprosy. Neurological signs are often present.

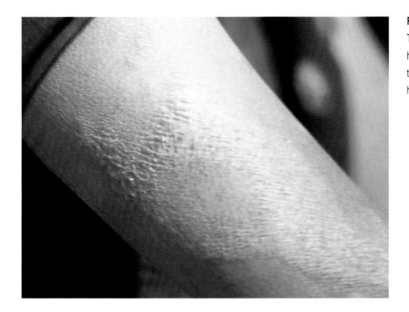

Fig. 5.5 Tuberculoid leprosy. The skin is dry, anaesthetic and hairless due to involvement of the sweat glands, nerves and hair follicles.

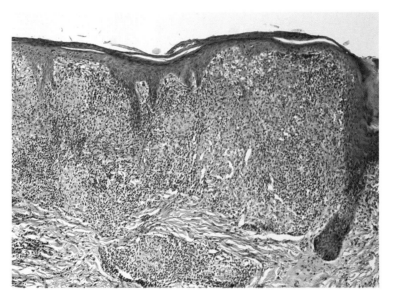

Fig. 5.6 Tuberculoid (TT) leprosy. Granulomata are eroding into the epidermis. No acid-fast bacilli are seen on Wade-Fite staining. By courtesy of Dr. S. Lucas, University College Hospital.

Lepromatous Leprosy

In this variety of leprosy the immunological response of the host is minimal. It is a widespread, progressive disease with bacilli invading not only the skin and nerves but also the reticuloendothelial system. The skin lesions are symmetrical and extensive, in contrast to those of tuberculoid leprosy. Neurological involvement occurs late in the disease, probably because the immunological response to the presence of the bacilli in the nervous tissue is minor and therefore little damage is done. The disease is highly infectious from nasal discharges, unlike tuberculoid leprosy which is not infectious at all.

The early cutaneous changes are often too subtle to be noticed by the patient. The first symptoms are usually nasal such as stuffiness, discharge and epistaxis. Swelling of the ankles and lower legs is common. The skin changes commence as symmetrical, small, red or slightly hypopigmented macules which are multiple and subsequently become extensive. They have vague and ill-defined borders. Anaesthetic

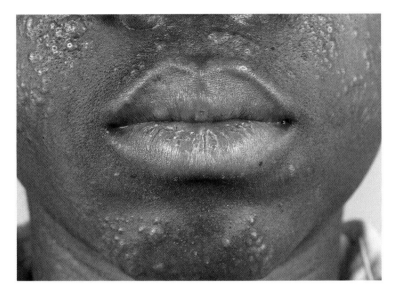

Fig. 5.7 Lepromatous leprosy. Extensive papules and nodules are present in this African. The lips are also involved.

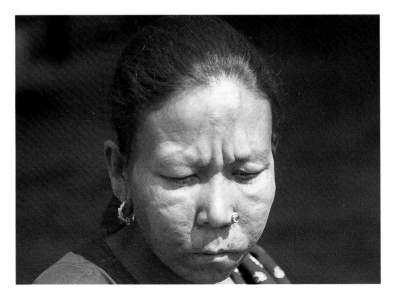

Fig. 5.8 Lepromatous leprosy. Diffuse infiltration of the face occurs.

papules, plaques and nodules (lepromata) develop later (Fig. 5.7). The face (Fig. 5.8), arms, legs and buttocks are characteristically affected but any area of the skin, other than warm sites such as the axillae and groin, may be involved. The cooler areas of the face, such as the lips, nose (Fig. 5.9) and earlobes (Figs. 5.10 and 5.11) are particularly involved. Diffuse infiltration of the skin of the forehead causes a

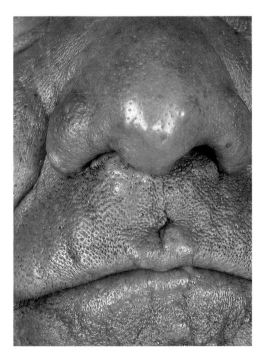

Fig. 5.9 Lepromatous leprosy. The nose and lips are characteristic sites.

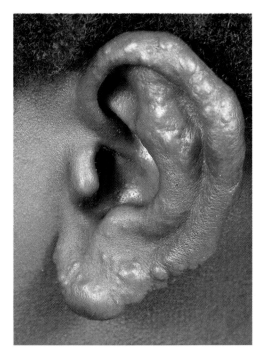

Fig. 5.10 Lepromatous leprosy. Papules and nodules around the ears are characteristic. Leprosy favours the peripheral areas of skin.

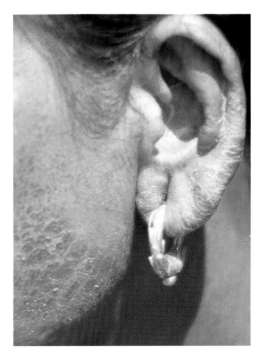

Fig. 5.11 Lepromatous leprosy. There is diffuse pink infiltration of the cheeks and ears.

leonine appearance (Fig. 5.12) and the eyebrows and eyelashes disappear. The nose, eyes, testes and bone become involved. Glove and stocking anaesthesia develops from polyneuritis (Fig. 5.13) and destruction and shortening of the digits result from frequent unappreciated trauma (Fig. 5.14). The course of the disease is punctuated by frequent febrile exacerbations and erythema nodosum leprosum is a characteristic feature. The untreated patient ultimately succumbs from renal failure or concomitant tuberculosis.

The diagnosis can be made by biopsy of the skin (Figs. 5.15 and 5.16). There are relatively few lymphocytes, but a large number of acid-fast bacilli are demonstrable in foamy, so-called 'lepra' cells. The diagnosis can also be made by making a superficial slit into involved skin and smearing the tissue thus gained onto a slide. This can be stained for acid-fast bacilli and the organisms demonstrated.

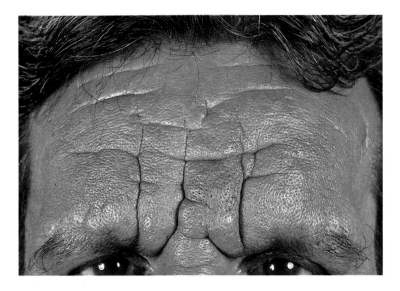

Fig. 5.12 Lepromatous leprosy. Involvement of the forehead has produced deep fissuring, so-called 'leonine facies'.

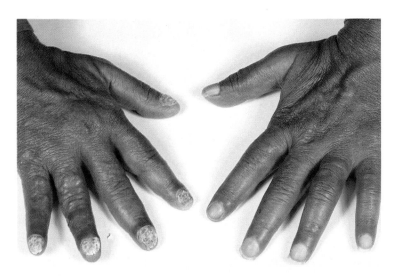

Fig. 5.13 Lepromatous leprosy, neuritis and tinea of the nails. Two lepromata are present on the fingers of the right hand. There is gross tinea of the nails secondary to immunosuppression. There is wasting of the small muscles of the hands.

The treatment of leprosy is the province of experts who have made the disease a life-long study. However, drugs such as dapsone, rifampicin and clofazimine have now turned this scourge of a disease into a treatable one.

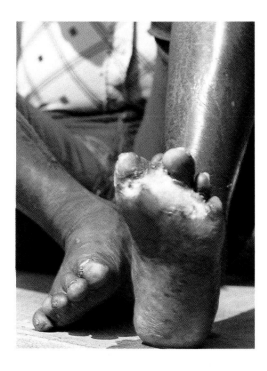

Fig. 5.14 Lepromatous leprosy. Destruction of the digits is an end result of glove and stocking anaesthesia.

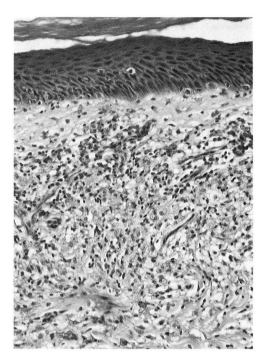

Fig. 5.15 Lepromatous leprosy. A diffuse infiltrate of foamy histiocytes (lepra cells) is separated from the epidermis by a grenz zone of sparing.

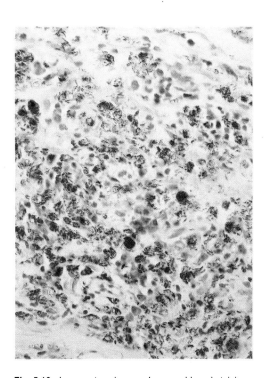

Fig. 5.16 Lepromatous leprosy. Innumerable red-staining bacilli may be demonstrated. The larger intracellular aggregates are sometimes known as globi. (Wade-Fite stain.)

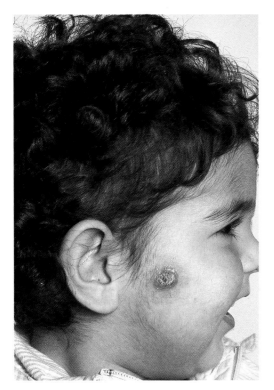
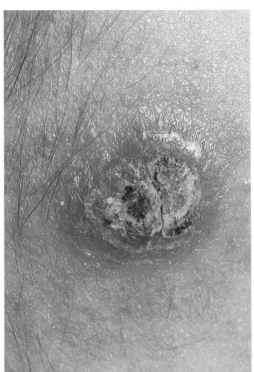

Fig. 5.17 Cutaneous leishmaniasis (Baghdad boil). This little boy was bitten on the face by an infected sandfly. The close-up shows a crusted ulcer.

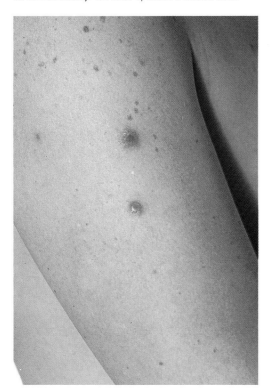
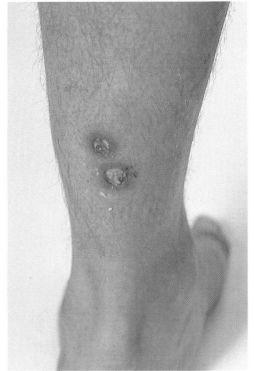

Fig. 5.18 Cutaneous leishmaniasis. This man received multiple infected sandfly bites whilst working in the Middle East. The initial lesions on the arm are red, slightly crusted papules. The red lesions on the legs have ulcerated and become indurated.

CUTANEOUS LEISHMANIASIS (Oriental Sore, Baghdad Boil)

This condition results from bites by sandflies infected with the protozoan, *Leishmania tropica*. It is common in the Middle East, subtropics and tropics, but also may occur in Mediterranean countries, especially North Africa, so it is increasingly encountered in holiday makers. The exposed parts (Fig. 5.17) are the most common sites to be bitten, resulting in papules and nodules which break down, ulcerate and crust (Figs. 5.18 and 5.19). They subsequently heal within a year, but with considerable

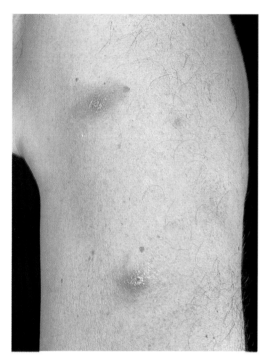 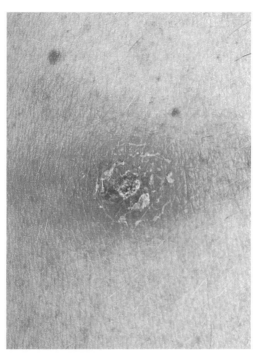

Fig. 5.19 Cutaneous leishmaniasis. Red nodules with a central crusted area are present.

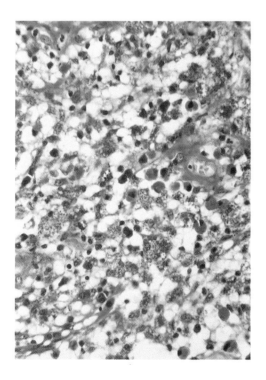

Fig. 5.20 Cutaneous leishmaniasis. The dermis is extensively infiltrated by large numbers of macrophages containing numerous *Leishmania* organisms. In addition, scattered, intensely eosinophilic Russell bodies are evident. The latter represent plasma cells distended by immunoglobulin.

scarring. The organism may be demonstrated in skin smears. Leishman Donovan bodies are seen within large histiocytes on skin biopsy (Fig. 5.20). Treatment with pentavalent antimony compounds may be effective.

LARVA MIGRANS

This is caused by hookworm larvae from the faeces of infected dogs. The condition occurs in the Caribbean and New World, and anyone walking barefoot or sitting on a contaminated beach is at risk. *Ancylostoma braziliensis* is the most common hookworm responsible. The site of entry (usually the buttocks or foot) is itchy at first and subsequently the patient notices a linear moving eruption (Figs. 5.21 and 5.22) which is intensely itchy and may become secondarily infected. The condition responds to topical application of thiabendazole.

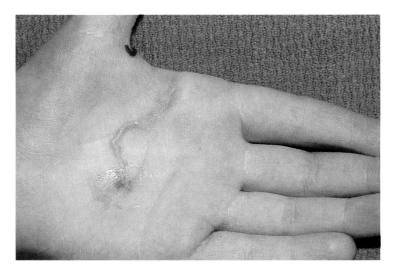

Fig. 5.21 Larva migrans. Linear mobile tracks occur. The disorder is due to canine hookworm larvae penetrating the skin.

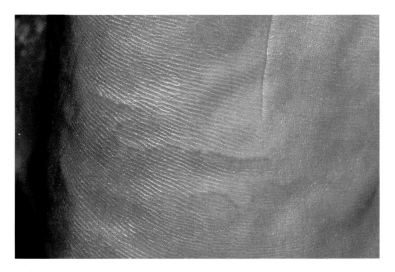

Fig. 5.22 Larva migrans. This man contracted this infection in his foot on a Caribbean beach where infected dogs roam free.

ONCHOCERCIASIS

This is an infestation with larvae of the roundworm *Onchocerca* (*Onchocerca volvulus* in Africa or *Onchocerca caecutiens* in Central America). Gnats (*Simuliidae*) transmit the disease by biting human skin and injecting the larvae, which then mature into worms and produce subcutaneous nodules. The condition is extremely pruritic and widespread papules and lichenification occur (Fig. 5.23) particularly around the shoulders and upper arms and buttocks and thighs. Microfilariae invade the dermis and destroy the elastic tissue so that the skin may hang in folds, especially in the groin. Scarring and pigmentary changes are frequent.

The most important consequence of the disease is invasion of the eye as it may result in blindness. The condition is known as 'river blindness' because the gnats breed close to rivers. The disorder is thus more likely to be contracted in rural rather than urban areas.

The microfilariae (Fig. 5.24) may be found by examining strips of skin in saline. There is frequently an eosinophilia and the filarial complement fixation test is positive. The disorder may be treated with diethylcarbamazine (Banocide) or suramin. Nodules may be excised.

BURULI ULCER

This is a tropical disease caused by *Mycobacterium ulcerans*. Buruli is a swampland district in Uganda. The organism is harboured by spiky grasses and can be inoculated into the bare legs of a passer-by. The

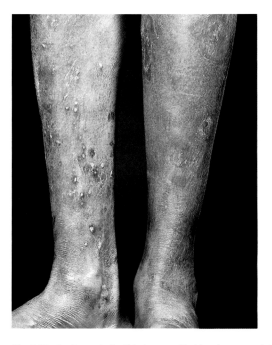 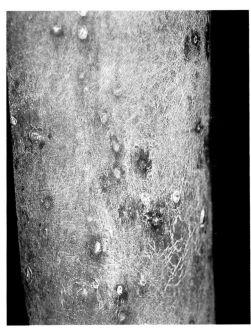

Fig. 5.23 Onchocerciasis. This is caused by bites from gnats infected with the larvae of the *Onchocerca* roundworm. The condition is extremely pruritic and widespread excoriated papules, lichenification and post-inflammatory hyperpigmentation occur. The skin is very dry. The lower limbs are comonly affected. By courtesy of Dr. Roger Clayton, St. Mary's Hospital.

condition is most often seen on the legs of young children. It presents as an ulcer with a deeply delineated edge (Fig. 5.25). The diagnosis is made by a skin biopsy and by culture of the organism from the skin. The condition does not respond to standard anti-tuberculous therapy and the ulcer needs to be widely excised and grafted as early as possible.

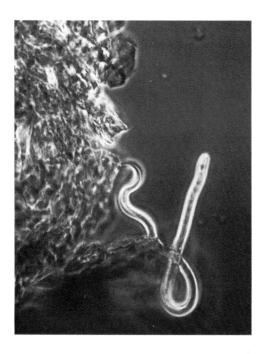

Fig. 5.24 Onchocerciasis. The microfilariae may be demonstrated in strips of skin in saline. By courtesy of Dr. Roger Clayton, St. Mary's Hospital.

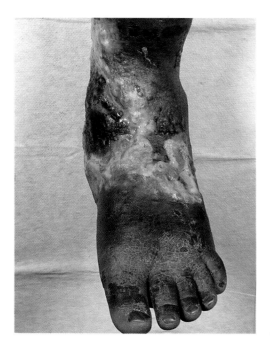
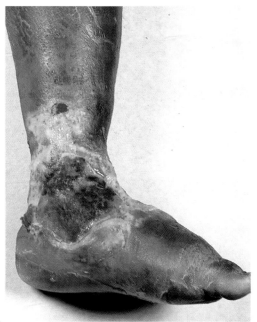

Fig. 5.25 Buruli ulcer. Children most commonly acquire this infection on the legs from contact with contaminated grasses. Extensive ulceration has occurred here and a large eschar is present. The condition is caused by *Mycobacterium ulcerans*. The infections must

be widely excised and grafted.

INDEX

E

ear, external *see* external ear
ecthyma 13
ectothrix infections 66–8
eczema
    atopic 38
    discoid 71–2
    herpeticum 38–9
    misdiagnosed as scabies 90
    predisposing to impetigo 4–5
    predisposing to molluscum
        contagiosum 50
eczematous eruption, caused by benzyl benzoate 92
elbows, scabies 88
encephalitis
    herpes simplex virus 38
    smallpox vaccination 44
endothrix infections 71
    tinea capitis 68–9
epidermis
    desquamation 15
    toxic necrolysis 14–15
Epidermophyton 65
    E. floccosum 75, 76, 77
erosio interdigitale 64
erysipelas 15–16
erysipeloid 17
Erysipelothrix rhusiopathiae 17
erythema
    induratum (Bazin's disease) 24–5
    multiforme
        herpes simplex infection 38
        orf 52
        smallpox vaccination 44
    nodosum 25
        leprosum 108
erythrasma 17–19
erythromycin
    erysipelas 16
    erythrasma 18
    staphylococccal impetigo 5
external ear
    involvement in herpes zoster 42
    otitis externa 9, 16
eyelashes, staphylococcal infection 12
eyes
    blindness, onchocerciasis 113
    infection
        herpes simplex 38
        herpes zoster 42–3
        pseudomonas folliculitis 9

F

face
    chronic mucocutaneous candidosis 65
    digitate warts 46
    erysipelas 15–16
    filiform warts 46
    folliculitis secondary to ingrowing hairs 8
    herpes simplex 36–9

face *(cont.)*
    impetigo 3
    lepromatous leprosy 106-7
    lupus vulgaris 20–1
    molluscum contagiosum 49
    plane warts 45
    primary tuberculosis of the skin 19
    secondary syphilis 30–1
    sycosis barbae 7–8
    tertiary syphilis 33
    tinea faciei 74
facial nerve palsy, herpes zoster 42
farmers, orf 51
favus 69
feet
    hand, foot and mouth disease 52–3
    plantar warts 46
    soles
        scabies 86–7
        secondary syphilis 30–31, 33
        Trichophyton rubrum infections 80
filiform warts 46–8
fingernails 81–3
fish-tank granuloma 26
fissuring, tinea pedis 77
fleas 95, 97
folliculitis 6–10
formalin 48
fumigation
    body lice 94
    ectoparasites 99
furunculosis (boils) 10–11

G

gamma benzene hexachloride 92–4
geniculate ganglion, herpes zoster 42
genitalia
    candida balanitis 63
    candidosis 62–3
    herpes simplex 36–9
    molluscum contagiosum 49
    primary syphilitic lesion 28
    scabies 89
    secondary syphilis 30–1, 33
    warts 46–8
gingivostomatitis, herpes simplex primary
  infection 36
glove and stocking anaesthesia 108–9
glucocorticosteroids *see* steroids
glycosuria, routine testing
    patients with boils 11
    patients with candida vaginitis 62–3
gnats 113
gonococcaemia 27
granulomata
    BCG 20
    fish-tank 26
    Majocchi's 80–1
    papulonecrotic tuberculide 25
    swimming pool 26
    tertiary syphilis 33
    tuberculoid leprosy 104–5

griseofulvin
   dermatophyte infections 83
   pityriasis versicolor 59
   tinea capitis 70, 72
groins
   candida intertrigo 63
   condylomata 31
   erythrasma 17–18
   tinea cruris 74–7
gummata 33–4

H

hair follicles
   bacterial infections 6–12
   pityriasis versicolor 56
hair loss *see* alopecia
hand, foot and mouth disease 52–3
hands
   chronic mucocutaneous candidosis 65
   common warts 44–5
   erysipeloid 17
   gonococcaemia 27
   hand, foot and mouth disease 52–3
   orf 52
   plane warts 45
   scabies 86
   tinea manuum 81, 83
Hansen's disease (leprosy) 102–9
head louse (pediculosis capitis) 92–3
   predisposing to impetigo 4
hepatitis, additional to secondary syphilis 30, 32
hepatosplenomegaly, congenital syphilis 34
hepatotoxicity, ketoconazole 59, 83
herpes simplex 36–9
herpes zoster (shingles) 40–4
herpetic whitlow 38
hexachlorophane 11
hirsutism
   Bockhart's impetigo 7
   crab lice 92
   keloids secondary to ingrowing hairs 8
   predisposing to folliculitis 10
homosexual men 28
hookworm larvae 112
hordeoli (styes) 12
horses 68
hot climates *see* tropical countries
Hutchinson's triad 34
hyperpigmentation
   pityriasis versicolor 56–8
   tinea corporis 72–3
   tinea cruris 76
hyphae 65, 69
hypopigmentation
   pityriasis versicolor 56–9
   tuberculoid leprosy 103

I

id phenomenon 78–9
idoxuridine in dimethyl sulphoxide
   herpes simplex 39
   herpes zoster 44
imidazole
   candida vaginitis 63
   dermatophyte infections 83
   erythrasma 18
   oral candidosis 60
   pityriasis versicolor 59
immunological reaction, papulonecrotic
   tuberculide 25
immunosuppression
   boils 11
   candidosis 60
   disseminated zoster 43
   herpes simplex virus 38–9
   herpes zoster 42–3
   Norwegian scabies 91
   tinea cruris 76
impetiginized eczema 4–5
impetigo 2–5
   Bockhart's 7
ingrowing hairs, secondary folliculitis 7–8
inoculation
   autoinoculation 3, 44
   spiky grasses, Buruli ulcer 113
insect bites 95–101
   cutaneous leishmaniasis 110–11
   ecthyma 13
insomnia, scabies 86
intertrigo
   candida intertrigo 63–4
   condylomata lata 31
   erythrasma 17–18
iodine, molluscum contagiosum 50
irradiation of tinea capitis 70, 72

J

jacuzzis—pseudomonas folliculitis 9
joints
   congenital syphilis 34
   gonococcaemia 27

K

Kaposi's varicelliform eruption 39
keloid formation
   folliculitis of the scalp 9
   secondary to ingrowing hairs 8
keratinophilic fungi 56
keratitis, herpes simplex 38
kerion 66–9, 71, 74